The Medical
COP-OUT

Cynthia Birrer

The Medical
COP-OUT

toExcel
San Jose New York Lincoln Shanghai

The Medical Cop-out

Published by toExcel
an imprint of iUniverse.com, Inc.

For information address:
iUniverse.com, Inc.
620 North 48th Street
Suite 201
Lincoln, NE 68504-3467
www.iuniverse.com

ISBN: 0-595-00606-X

Printed in the United States of America

Acknowledgments

To my mother and father, to my friends, the big ones and the little ones, to those few doctors who did not let the side down: thank you.

To the men and women with multiple sclerosis, and to the others who shared their experiences of pain with me: my gratitude.

To Professor Strauss, for his intellectual integrity and academic acumen: my admiration. Needless to say, however, the views I have expressed - legal or otherwise - are not necessarily shared by Professor Strauss.

To the editorial staff of Human & Rousseau, for their courtesy and considerable assistance: my appreciation.

To Ivan Illich, for the will to self-determination, to endure and to grow: my return.

for
BILL
husband, friend and mentor

"Our legal system is strange and awesome, a fumbling, imponderable leviathan. That it often achieves a semblance of justice is remarkable. As might be said of medicine, it is the most workable system, for the nature of the social needs it serves, that human ingenuity has, as yet, been able to contrive. Let us hope, nevertheless, that creative thinkers will continue tirelessly searching for means to improve, reform, remodel and refine it."

HERBERT C. MODLIN, M.D.

Contents

Prologue

S. A. Strauss
Professor of Law, University of South Africa

For millennia men in search of solutions to their most pressing problems have knocked on the doors of three types of professional men in particular: the physician, the priest and the lawyer. In primitive societies the roles of the medicine man, the prophet-priest and the lawmaker-jurist were probably indistinguishable. But as society developed these areas of professionalism tended to diverge. Today they are distinctly separate, and together with a host of other specialist and technical disciplines they serve modern industrial man.

But the physician's skill is still one of the most sought after of all. Of all the ancient professional fields, his has now undoubtedly become the most unrecognizable as compared to its older manifestations. But it has been said that natural science is modern man's religion, and in so far as this is true, the doctor's image has perhaps again become more closely identifiable with that of the priest.

In his more primitive role, the physician was admired for his apparent access to the mysteries of the supernatural world, coupled with his knowledge of the human body. In his modern guise, he is held in almost religious awe because of his knowledge and utilization of the vast array of technical skills and pharmaceutical products put at his disposal by modern science.

Much has been said about the marvels of modern medicine. In fact, the modern reader, listener and viewer is fed on a constant diet of facts and fiction relating to doctors and medicine. As humanity was battered by one catastrophe after the other – pestilence and plague, drought and famine, insurrection, terrorism and war, the spectre of overpopulation – the medical scientist became one of the most hopeful beacons of light in a dark and sinister universe. The utter adulation with which most of mankind regarded the men who performed the first heart transplants is symbolic of man's intrinsic faith in modern medicine.

As was the case in primitive societies where mysticism reigned

11

supreme, man has again become conditioned to expect miracles from the médical man. There seems to be no end to what modern science can provide.

If the doctor is perhaps more realistic than laymen about the range of his therapeutic capabilities, he is certainly no less impressed by the seemingly endless series of spectacular aids emerging from modern chemistry and technology, and he has displayed great enthusiasm for testing and utilising these.

But there is also a danger in this. Medicine, in the words of Paul Ferris, author of *The Doctors,* is "putting its future firmly in the hands of scientists and mathematicians, who are never far from machines, laboratories and the dynamics of shared experience". As the technological aids come to the fore, the human being behind them is inclined to recede into the background. Many of us - as patients - have had the experience of going through a complicated series of diagnostic checks and techniques, with nothing more than a fleeting glance - perhaps in semi-darkness - of the specialist himself. It is common experience for patients to undergo surgery without seeing the surgeon in the operating theatre. Leading doctors have often warned about the communication gap in the modern doctor-patient relationship.

Yet, with all its aura of science and technology, medicine is still regarded as more of an art than a science. But has the super-technology of our time, coupled with the veneration of the medical profession by the man in the street, not perhaps had the effect that doctors on occasion underestimate their own fallibility?

I raise this question in all humility. As a patient, and also as a lawyer with a more than passing interest in forensic medicine and medical law, I share in the almost universal admiration of the medical profession. Like millions of other people, my family and I have experienced the tremendous benefits which flow from modern medicine. We are grateful for these. We place great trust in the doctors whom we consult and who attend to us with such skill and compassionate care. Already I am tactfully encouraging my son, eight years of age now, to become a doctor one day - although I must say that the appearance of the *Chopper One* series on television seems to have rekindled his original enthusiasm for a career in the police force.

Nonetheless, even in full appreciation of the benefits of modern medicine and of science in general, one is acutely aware of the gradual process of "de-personalization" affecting so many areas of our lives in this scientific age. It is of course not confined to the practice of medicine. During a recent visit of three months to Germany my house was firmly locked all the time. But my telephone accounts, forwarded to Germany by my secretary, kept indicating calls being registered on my number. In order not to have my service terminated, I faithfully paid the accounts, intending to take up the matter with the Post Office on my return. This I did, arguing – convincingly, I thought – that I was physically away for three months, that no one had access to my house, and that I had found no signs of forcible entry into my residence. But the Post Office blandly responded that I have no cause of action: their computer cannot be wrong. I gave up the battle without having really commenced it.

Some readers might wish to write off Cynthia Birrer's book as a crusade against the medical profession by a patient who has become embittered on account of having expected more from medicine than she ought to have. It is nothing of the sort. We have here a very articulate and at times poignant account of the experiences of a person who, like countless others, has sought an explanation for terrifying symptoms which suddenly assailed her body. She sought assistance from those who could possibly help her, the doctors. If her book is critical of the actions and attitudes of some doctors, it to an equal extent praises the actions and attitudes of others.

Cynthia Birrer asked me to write the foreword to her book in the form of a prologue. In doing so I shall not endeavour to pass judgment on any of the medical *dramatis personae* of this work. As a lawyer trained in the spirit of *audi alteram partem,* I would not venture to do so unless I have had the advantage of hearing the other side as well. I do therefore not take sides. All I want to say is that in her book Cynthia Birrer has touched upon several raw nerves in the present system of adjudication of medical malpractice suits. If her book is seen as being critical of the medical profession, it is to an equal extent an indictment of the inadequacies of our legal system.

The privilege of being a doctor or a lawyer brings awesome responsibilities for those who put up their shingles. Both doctor and lawyer must probe deeply into facts, make findings and take action which might subsequently have a profound effect on the lives of the people who put themselves into their hands. Speaking on behalf of my own profession, the law, we can never afford to be smug or content with either our legal system, or the practices of our profession.

As lawyers we should always be self-critical and prepared to suffer public scrutiny. We are practising our profession not only for our own sakes, but above all to provide a service to the community. We should avoid being unduly sensitive to criticism coming from our clients or ex-clients, or from the public at large.

In my experience of the medical profession, this certainly is the attitude of the vast majority of doctors. The spirit of utter self-sacrifice which many doctors display and the way in which the South African Medical and Dental Council supervises the professional and ethical standards of doctors can serve as an example to other professional groups.

Yet, because Cynthia Birrer has exposed sensitive nerves, she must expect a reaction to her book, perhaps even a vehement reaction. Professional groups can be very sensitive to such exposures. In particular, any mention of what the Americans have termed the "conspiracy of silence" in regard to a professional group is like waving a scarlet cape to the face of a well-trained, battle-keen Castilian bull.

During 1976 I was requested to participate in a popular discussion programme on medical liability broadcast on Radio South Africa. My co-participant was one of the most eminent medical doctors of this country. Our discussion was, so I thought, in the nature of a rather low-key conversation. At one stage, having outlined the very real difficulties which patients experience in obtaining expert medical evidence in bringing legal action for alleged malpractice, I referred in very guarded terms to the impression one gains of the so-called "conspiracy of silence" in some professional groups, inter alia the medical profession. My co-participant on the programme seemed to agree conditionally with me in the following terms: "Yes, perhaps there is a sort of – I do not know whether the word 'brotherhood' can actually be applied here – but the sort of thing that one knows, well, I am exposed, so all right, we have to protect each other a bit. I must confess that I am not clearly aware of such a thing. I do not often hear my colleagues talk among themselves in these terms. But that it may perhaps exist in fact – that I will concede. However, what does occur, is that my colleagues in fact frequently experience problems in giving evidence in court . . ." The doctor then proceeded to describe the practical difficulties which medical men experience in acting as witnesses, such as disruption of their practices, financial loss, waste of time, etc.

14

In the course of the radio programme I observed that the standard of medical practice in South Africa was of the highest in the world, and that doctors as a professional group were probably less negligent than others. I also expressed the opinion – based on my own experience and that of colleagues – that not one out of a hundred cases of alleged medical malpractice in which lawyers were consulted ended up in the courts. I said that there were several reasons for this, two of them being the difficulties for the plaintiff to discharge the onus of proof resting on him, and the problems experienced by lawyers to obtain medical witnesses to testify for the plaintiff. The Medical Association reacted almost immediately to my observations, doing me the rare honour of issuing a 1 500-word rebuttal, in polite but stern terms, in the form of a special loose-leaf insert in the *South African Medical Journal.*

It was with keen interest that I read in the Association's statement that its Federal Council had resolved to appoint a panel of medical experts to be at the disposal of the Medical Council and courts of law when expert evidence was required. However, the General Secretary of the Association was at pains to point out that this was not because of the alleged reluctance of doctors to testify, but because of "the fact that so often conflicting expert opinions are aired during court trials". Regardless of why such a panel is being instituted, no one will be more enthusiastic about it than Cynthia Birrer.

Perhaps I should repeat here what I said in a paper (to which Mrs. Birrer also makes reference in her book) read at the First World Meeting on Medical Law which was held at the University of Ghent, Belgium, in 1967: Lawyers are inclined to lay the blame for the difficulty of securing an expert medical witness to testify for the plaintiff squarely at the door of the medical profession. The most extreme view is that there is a "conspiracy of silence" among medical men. But this view hardly deserves serious attention. It is manifestly unjust to the medical profession to brand physicians as cold-blooded members of an esoteric brotherhood who are deliberately pledged to silence for their mutual benefit, without the slightest regard for the interests of patients who suffer as a result of lack of skill or inadvertence on the part of their doctors. There is undoubtedly a spirit of cameraderie among physicians, but to indicate this as the root of the trouble amounts to an oversimplification. The reason for the problem, I said, lies partially in forensic procedures. There are, of course, physicians who do not hesitate to come forward as witness for the plaintiff, as is also borne out by many reported decisions in favour of plaintiffs. However, I stressed, whatever the reasons may be, finding an expert medical witness does present an initial obstacle to many a prospective plaintiff whose complaint is genuine.

Cynthia Birrer has highlighted this unsolved dilemma in the administration of justice. The difference is that while lawyers and doctors discuss the problem *in abstracto,* to her as a patient and client it is something very real and very personal. Her thoughts on it are stimulating and thought-provoking. But the reader will note that her thinking goes beyond the immediate issue of individual accountability. As she points out, it ultimately becomes a matter of collective liability.

This brief prologue would not be complete without some personal reference to the author of this book. Cynthia Birrer is a remarkable person. In a way her book can be subtitled "an autobiography of suffering". An autobiography can, of course, never be objective. As is apparent from her book, her experiences must have generated deep emotion towards the personalities and situations involved. Yet she has related her experiences in the spirit of an invitation to the reader to judge the nature of a human relationship rather than the characters of those involved. Her story is of necessity an intimate one and she has written it with sensitivity. Her irrepressible humour and persistent courage in the face of great adversity and physical pain will serve as an example to all of us.

Pretoria,
July, 1976

Preface

This story is true. The identities of the doctors concerned in the case have been concealed, but I have set down all the other facts in some detail, as carefully and as objectively as possible, having regard to my role as the patient. There is no statement in the following pages that cannot be corroborated. Even my difficulties in making contact with the specialist in charge of the case were witnessed by one friend or another.

I have chosen to keep the exposition short and to the point, eliminating details of personality that perhaps might have added a dimension of "human interest", whatever that may mean, but that would also have blurred the central intention, namely that what has been written will spark off responsible debate on the grave moral, social, medical and legal issues which the entire conduct of the case raises. I have used the case, and my earlier medical history, not so much to tell my story, but as pegs on which to hang the questions that emerge in the circumstances of alleged medical malpractice.

I am concerned with general principles, and not with any particular instance, because it is clear from many discussions with men in both the medical and legal professions that the case, while unique in detail, represents a phenomenon that is virtually a weekly occurrence. In essence, therefore, it is an example, or model, and the reader is invited to regard it as a slim document on which to form a judgment, not on the characters of those involved, although this factor is certainly not purely incidental, but on whether the nature of the relationship which presently exists in South Africa between the doctor, the patient and the law is equitable and satisfactory. If the answer is that it is not, and that the sick are in effect a perniciously exploited minority group, steps must be taken to excise, and to apply a remedy for, this most malignant social cancer.

I returned, and saw under the sun, that the race is not to the swift, nor the battle to the strong, neither yet bread to the wise, nor yet riches to men of understanding, nor yet favour to men of skill; but time and chance happeneth to them all. For man also knoweth not his time; as the fishes that are taken in an evil net, and as the birds that are caught in the snare; so are the sons of men snared in an evil time, when it falleth suddenly upon them.

ECCLESIASTES 9, 11-12

Part I Mistaken Identity

1

It was nearly the end of 1973 before I was willing to admit, even to myself, that I was not well. But the day dawned when the physical and psychological changes that had so insidiously been permeating my consciousness for some time could no longer be ignored. I felt that I knew exactly *what* was happening, from the physical point of view. The sequence of events and my experience of them was quite specific and easy to detail, even though the web of underlying circumstance was so insubstantial that I pushed it far back into the recesses of my mind. Psychologically, too, I was aware of what was going on. But I had not even the suspicion of an idea as to why. I had read nothing that could throw a glimmer of light on the apparent metamorphosis I was undergoing - obvious not only to myself, but to those who knew me well.

At the beginning, in the opening months of 1974, I thought that perhaps something in the social environment was responsible: maybe it was an unconscious striving to shed a life-style, as a chrysalis sheds a cocoon. Whatever it was, my attitudes were undergoing a radical transformation. The most clearly definable aspect of this surrealist deformation of character was, quite simply, that I had ceased to care. I had replaced empathic concern by a state of absolute insensitivity to the other, a degenerate and devastating numbness of mind. This was not only my subjective experience; it was an objective fact, a phenomenon as painfully real as it was grotesque. At first I regarded it with mild surprise, then with deep puzzlement and later, particularly in the early months of 1975, with alarm and despondency. By that time I was sure I had undergone an irreversible dissolution of personality. In a few short months I had become exactly the kind of person I abhor: totally uninvolved in anything at all, unmoved and unmovable, with no regard for the past, no sense of rootedness in the present and a total unconcern for the morrow, no matter what it may bring. Divorce, death, damnation were not merely trivia; they no longer had any meaning whatever for me.

This debauchery was a denial of the leitmotiv of my life: an insatiable fascination with the human condition. Now I did not care about my husband, my parents, my home, my friends, my beloved pets – or my job, which was lecturing in developmental and cognitive psychology in the Department of Education at the University of the Witwatersrand. I wanted to turn my back, slamming every door behind me, and walk away from life without a backward glance. And this, in effect, is exactly what I did. I packed my bags, deserted my home, shook off familial responsibility and began to live alone. I withered in other respects too; my compassion for the victims of job reservation and pass laws and the migratory labour system, and my deep disgust and despair at the consequent arbitrary abolition of family life vanished, as my own behaviour so vividly confirmed. I felt no necessity to justify my actions, but I tried to do so out of a last vestige of pity for those whose lives I was heedlessly bludgeoning into the ground: I needed complete privacy, seclusion from an environment that had become irrelevant, isolation from people who had become redundant, in order to sort out the reasons for my own psychological demission, reasons which eluded rational analysis. I had taken the suicidal plunge into the dank slime of a moral void, seemingly without rhyme or legitimate reason.

I was as aware as I had always been of social issues, I listened as intently as I always had to discussions and arguments around them, I made the noises people had come to expect from me, but I felt nothing. Circumstances and events washed over me, and – like the incoming tide on a sandy beach – receded and left no impress.

Only once was I jarred by my state of affective anaesthesia. I have long refused to set foot in a certain Johannesburg private club because of its policy of restricted membership. But in June of 1974, when I was reluctantly obliged to plan a rather large cocktail party, I suggested this club as a venue. Bill, my husband, regarded me in wide-eyed astonishment.

"But you won't go near the place!" he exclaimed incredulously.

"Oh, well, what does it matter – who cares, anyway?"

It was shocking, and anyone who knew me well would have been shocked. More than that, I think they would have denied the very possibility that I could adopt such an attitude. I began to fear the moral and emotional bankruptcy that loomed before me. I know that common candour regarding civil, social, economic and political inequity among the peoples of South Africa requires uncommon courage, but I also know that the price we are paying for our apathy, our guilt by neglect, is even higher. Somewhere along the line the rot sets in and we begin to reflect, each in his own way, the dominant values of the greater society. What I did not know, what I did not remotely suspect, was just how great that cost really is, and how far the erosion has spread. It is impossible to imagine that the same ruthless perversion of human values could characterise the professional behaviour and attitudes of some of Johannesburg's foremost doctors. But that was exactly what I found. It became terrifyingly apparent during the conduct of my case in the first eleven months of 1975 that the Hippocratic Oath, which is the most impressive document in medical ethics and which has been administered to medical graduates at European universities for centuries, can be as feeble and futile as many of the other checks and balances forged in the crucible of Western civilisation to safeguard the humanitarian ideal.

The emotional debilitation I felt was echoed by the real fatigue of my body. I was generally fatigued, waking tired in the morning, going to bed in a state of exhaustion. But there was also fatigue that was induced by specific activities: walking, driving back and forth, climbing stairs in particular, all this sort of thing tired me. The tiredness was exacerbated by some odd difficulties with my right leg. After walking even short distances I often found that I literally could not take another step with it. There was no pain, but if I pushed myself beyond this limit the leg dragged badly. Fortunately it soon recovered with rest, but its annoying quirk considerably limited how much I was able to do each day. The knee was a problem, too: there was consistent, though not unbearable pain in it, and it had the frequent and disconcerting habit of giving way, almost as if in response to pressure on the sole of the foot. I kept tripping over my own feet and sometimes I fell, twice in the street. I did not know how I came to be there, I was not conscious of the knee reneging or of stumbling, .but there I was, sitting on my bottom in the middle of the pavement. Walls and doors on my right acted like a magnet; I bumped into them, over and over again, and into low tables and the sharp corners of desks, always leading with the right side, so that upper arm and thigh and shin were seldom completely free of bruises.

The leg was also troublesome on waking. I learned to open my eyes, keep still, and move only very slowly. Nevertheless, as soon as I rolled onto my right side, or stretched the leg towards the bottom of the bed, spasms would convulse the calf, and the toes would ache with a violent cramp that forced them downward. The spasms were intensely painful and seldom abated within fifteen to twenty minutes. When I was at home, Bill often had to help me with massage or hot water bottles. I cannot remember a single morning during 1974 when the spasms did not occur, although once I was up and about there was no recurrence. I did have severe cramp on the odd occasion when I woke during the night and moved my legs around. I also learned to avoid sitting too far back in a chair or crossing my legs, at the knees or below, since doing this had the tendency either to put my right foot to sleep or to set off sharp bouts of pins and needles, sometimes in both feet.

Physically and emotionally I was enervated and apathetic. Surprisingly, though, the rapid devastation of my affective life did not find much violent overt expression. Sometimes, though not often, I experienced mild irritation, which I was able to suppress. On only three occasions in the fifteen months between January 1974 and March 1975 did I lash out. The first time was in January 1974, at Bill. I threw the book at him, everything that had happened during our married life that I viewed with disfavour, in microscopic detail, whether he was responsible directly, indirectly or not at all. I screamed like a shrew and left the house immediately afterwards. In June of that year something similar occurred. This time there was slightly more cause for a temperamental outburst, as I was involved in preparations for a conference which drained me completely. I exploded with a wrath quite disproportionate to the aggravation, venting my spleen on an older woman whom I had always greatly respected. The last time I exploded was in March 1975, when for no really good reason I ordered a friend out of my life, with explicit instructions to stay out. I do not remember whether I actually said that I did not care whether he lived or died, but it was certainly the way I felt. During the course of a private soliloquy afterwards I assured myself that the gentleman had manipulated my plainly anomolous situation rather nicely to his own selfish advantage, giving nothing of himself in return, so that he had really asked for all he got, which was plenty. On each of these occasions I knew exactly what I was doing, and I was also perfectly aware of the dire distress it caused in my listeners, but I felt not a twinge of remorse.

However, despite the lassitude of spirit and lethargy of body, I was often euphoric: I felt invulnerable, I felt an intense sense of mental vigour. It was this curious paradox that got me going and kept me going during 1974. I was expanding by leaps and bounds my knowledge of the psychology of infancy, an area I had not been directly concerned with before. I began to formulate a hitherto unexplored approach to an understanding of the pre-verbal child. The work was extremely demanding, requiring mastery of many skills in new areas before I could make headway. Nothing seemed too difficult; in fact, nothing *was* too difficult. I was continually amazed by the ease and speed with which I was able to penetrate a problem and recognise the direction in which to move for answers. It was obvious that if the theory I was working on evolved cogently enough, it could provide a novel and fruitful perspective on early human development. Fifteen leading pediatricians, psychologists, psychiatrists and biologists at universities in England and America agreed to co-operate in a symposium, the results of which should be published in 1977, in a combined effort to further the enterprise. In addition, I completed a long integrative monograph of pediatric and psychological research on the early mother-child relationship, and this was accepted for publication without modification by a professional journal in America.

They were strange, strange days: physically and emotionally depleted, I was nevertheless attempting intellectual gymnastics that would have quelled a more seasoned researcher with unlimited funds and bibliographic material at his disposal. And what was more, I was succeeding. Under the circumstances I would have forced myself to carry on without seeking medical assistance, had it not been for the growing impetus of another untoward development which had manifested itself early in 1974.

2

I had my first bout of double vision in January 1974. I was in a book shop studying the shelves when the objects in front of me began to peel apart. It was the first in a long series of attacks, and although their frequency varied from once in eight to ten days to only once or twice in three weeks, their form did not. They were always preceded by a short period during which I felt very ill. Then there was a "vee-ing" sensation: that is, the split would yield two images of the same object at the top, but only a single image at the base. The separation would become complete within a few seconds, resulting in two distinct images at some distance from each other on the horizontal plane; subjectively, I had the impression that if I moved forward I could pass between them. They retained their clarity, their colour and dimensionality for approximately fifteen minutes, when they would become misty and muted, and appear to exist on a flat surface; I was looking at a canvas that was distinctly concave at the centre. This impression would last a short while before the images fused again. At that point I would move unsteadily, falling sidewards easily and banging into everything while I concentrated on positioning my feet. Within about half an hour my head would seem numb. One of two things then followed: either I got a headache in my eyes, which ached on rotation, and if I pressed on the closed lids with my fingers, there was some pain; or else I experienced pain over the top of my head, an even, deadened effect with no throb. In both cases I had then to sleep for a long period. As the attacks never occurred after 11 a.m., this meant until the next morning. Sometimes I woke for dinner, but more often I did not feel like eating, although I was never nauseous. Sleep was imperative: I simply cancelled my classes for the day and left the campus.

That was my long-distance double vision, but there were also difficulties at closer range when reading or writing, particularly in artificial light. This was a huge problem to me until treatment of the disease began in December 1975: the rising and falling of oncoming headlights drove me wild, the "flicker" mechanism of the EEG, like a candle, could induce great agitation, and sitting for any length of time in a brightly lit auditorium was well-nigh impossible. Doing book work induced patchy vision; the centre portion of the print would lose its inky gloss, become greyish and within seconds bleach out entirely. Some print would be visible on the periphery, more at the top and bottom than on the sides. However, when the middle came back into focus, the remainder would patch out. This alternation would persist for variable lengths of time. When it was short-lived, I was generally left with a mild headache and blurring in the right eye. I tried to clear this by slitting the eye, tugging gently at the outside corner. When it was of longer duration, my right hand would begin to tremble. If I was writing at the time, the trembling could travel up the arm into the right shoulder and then, somehow, affect the left arm very slightly. The upper limbs felt extremely weak, and the right hand tremble and arm shake usually continued until I went to bed, feeling thoroughly squeamish. I retched once or twice, a horrid, tearing experience.

My right hand often trembled on exertion, sometimes when I did nothing more than lift a cup of tea or brush my hair, so much so that I broke an enduring childhood rule: one hundred strokes with the brush morning and evening. But its most upsetting effect usually occurred when I had to carry anything. Even carrying a heavy book a short distance to the library presented problems. Regardless of whether I held this at my side, pressed hard into the thigh, or shifted it from right hand to left, or cradled it in both arms, the trembling would be present when I set the book down. I would then not be able to write at all for about half an hour, and after that only a spidery, illegible hand. My writing did not return to normal in less than five hours. My mother, who proofed my manuscripts with me, remarked more than once on the considerable deterioration in my handwriting.

Today, the little finger and ring finger of my right hand tingle incessantly, unless both are numb; however, there is the complication of a short scar from a shallow but jagged cut in the inner edge of the wrist. In any event, objects continually slip out of my hand, and I am not aware of this until I hear the clatter. Wise friends who value their crockery have long since learned not to hand me a cup and saucer; these, as well as dinner plates, are tactfully set down in front of me.

Some time during March 1974 I noticed that my right eyelid was drooping badly and that the pupil was tightly constricted, whereas the left one was often fully dilated. Here again it was not until treatment began in December of the following year that the eyelid returned firmly to normal and the pupils equalised. The first day that it was obvious that this was definitely so I virtually spent in front of the mirror - I quite literally could not believe the evidence of my own eyes. But that March I could only console myself with the reminder of an elderly French actress who does not seem to worry in the least about her severe ptosis. She is a remarkable combination of noblesse oblige, haute couture and Kenneth Clark's *Civilisation,* and would look quite wrong without the drooping eyelid and half-closed eye. However, the role was a bit beyond me then, so I adopted a few tactics that disguised the defect - assuming a position just below my companion's shoulders, for example, squatting on table tops or chair arms, which also took the weight off my leg. This way I could always look up, so that the ptosis was less noticeable. Moreover, in this position my vision was clearer than when I looked downwards or glanced to either side.

Anyway, my positioning tactics must have worked – that or the increasingly skilful use of heavy make-up – because it was not until October that my ptosis was first mentioned. A friendly neurologist even went so far as to ask why I didn't wash all that muck off my face, I didn't need it, I wasn't old enough. If the boys who know all about these things overlooked it – well, I thought, it could not be so bad. It was a long time before the weight of accumulating evidence forced me to acknowledge the frightening frequency with which these men fall short of an immaculate perception. But then, it is well said that there are none so blind as those who will not see.

At the very end of September 1974 I returned home late one evening after a lecture. I poured myself a sherry and sat down at my desk to make a few notes. Instead I studied the amber liquid and began to think about myself: so much seemed to be running amok that I could not put my finger on. I mulled over the emotional somnolence, the souped-up mental machinery, the increasing fatigue in the lower limbs and weakness in the upper – and my sight. I worried about an attack of long-distance double vision I had had while driving. There had been an untimely fit, too.

Bill and I had dined in a restaurant and then moved on to the theatre. I got out of the car, but as I took each step the leading foot shot sideways with a sharp, spastic jerk. Bill gripped me under the right armpit.

"For goodness sake, what are you doing? You look quite drunk."

About an hour after we were seated I thought it was going to be an attack of double vision. The stage dimmed, but it kept its unity. I felt faint. Out in the foyer, I stopped suddenly, my head dropped backwards, eyes open, and I keeled over stiffly to the right.

Something similar had happened the previous month, at a cinema. But I had ignored both events, since I had had a few fits and faints some years before, and these had vanished as abruptly as they had appeared.

I did not know what to do or where to turn. There was Ann, a friend of very long standing, but she was so baffled by the little she had seen of the situation that neither of us would probably have made much sense of it. Then there was a particular friend on the university staff, but he was at the time so preoccupied with other matters that I could not expect a constructive hearing there, either. In fact, I had no reason to think that anyone would understand the kaleidoscopic pattern into which my existence had shattered.

I contemplated the situation and finally decided to go to an ophthalmologist. It was as good a place to start as any – and surely the one where the least harm could be done. I made an appointment for 22nd October, 1974, with Gerald Davids, whom I knew slightly through my work at the university.

Davids greeted me warmly at the door of the consulting room. I sat down in his resplendent chair as we chatted about the stress of the year-end examinations for the students in medical school. Maybe an open-book system was the best alternative. No, he didn't think so; that isn't the way it is done in America, and post-graduates from that country are generally of the highest calibre, study-wise at any rate. I agreed. I was also wondering why he was prolonging the conversation when outside his waiting room resembled a blown sardine can.

"Cynthia, how long has your eyelid been like that?"

"I'm not sure, really. I noticed it in March."

He paced across the room and turned back to me. "How do you feel – generally, you know, in yourself?"

I hesitated. "I don't feel very well. I'm so listless and everything has become such a sweat. But I'm most worried about my eyes – I've even thought that I might lose the right one."

"Do you see double?"

"Yes, often."

He sat down and carefully examined my eyes. "Well, I'm not worried about your sight – for distance, anyway, you prefer your own eyes. But I don't like that eyelid. Are you on your own?"

"If you mean did I come here on my own, yes."

"Can someone bring you tomorrow? I want to give you a shot of Tensilon, but I would prefer you not to drive immediately afterwards."

"Not tomorrow. Monday."

"Fine. Any time after 5 p.m."

Bill was with me when I had the injection. Gerald studied the right eye closely. According to him the eyelid shot up, a very positive reaction. I waited until the ghastly taste left my mouth. "Well?"

"I think you may have myasthenia."

27

So that was why he had used Tensilon. If the introduction of this drug intravenously increases the muscular power of the failing part (and the positive response of my eyelid showed that it did), then it is likely that the weakness in this part is myasthenic. Muscular weakness may be symptomatic of something else, but I was not sure if that was what Davids thought. I put out a feeler.

"Me and Onassis?"

"Yes." He grinned. "You're in good company."

Ouch. Onassis was badly affected by myasthenia gravis, a disease in which the muscles innervated by the cranial nerves, especially those connected with the eyes, are usually the first to suffer. Later the muscles of the neck, limbs and trunk become involved. I looked at Davids, waiting now for the good news.

He touched my arm lightly. "I want you to see a neurologist."

"No chance - no ways."

"Don't talk nonsense. I haven't the equipment necessary to do further tests. If you have myasthenia, you'll feel a different person under treatment."

"A neurologist - like who?"

"Bruce Green."

"But is he any good? You're talking about my nervous system - I want the *best*."

"He is."

"All right. But I'd like to make a few inquiries first."

I did. I solicited the opinions of several doctors, and they unanimously acclaimed Green's neurological expertise. I phoned his surgery.

"I'm afraid the first available appointment is 20th December. Dr. Green is very busy."

"Oh. All right." As long as the man knew what he was doing, it was worth waiting two months. "Will you let me know if there is a cancellation, please?" Once I had made up my mind, better sooner than later.

3

A friend drove me to the surgery when the fateful day came round. As I faced the man who was being entrusted with - above all things - my brain, many thoughts passed through my mind. I had been reluctant, now I was resigned. Seventeen years before the course of my life had been radically altered by an experience that had starkly emphasised the massive element of chance in medical practice. There was a second experience as well, a year later, that still rankled. I gazed and gazed at this doctor and wondered.

He looked Jewish. I thought about my first marriage, at the age of twenty, to a Jew - one of those who did *not* become a doctor. The marriage was opposed by his family and by my own, but we prevailed in the end. Our time together was brief, but it became a dominant force in my life. I loved my Jew and tried to grasp what it was that made him seem so different from the other men I knew. He gave me an insight into the basic tenets of the Jewish faith, so that when the pain of our parting had passed, I saw life differently. My growing involvement with Judaism reversed the aimless drift of a happy but frivolous adolescence, encouraging and nourishing in me an enduring love of learning - something which anxious parents and irate teachers alike had failed to do. My career as an academic began to take shape, and I always remember with deep affection the joyous association in which one strand of it is rooted.

I began to feel a bit better about things and cheered up. Expert medical skill wedded to the positive humanistic values intrinsic to Judaism, and to the spirit and ethic of the noble art of medicine, promised success. Many months were to slip by before I came to realise that this holy alliance had not been forged. But at that particular moment the thought uppermost in my mind was that he should do his job properly. There was no way of telling whether he would. I had held out for the best and I had been assured that this august presence was the very embodiment of neurologic excellence, and there was nothing more I could do on that score.

There were several factors I wanted to stress. First of all, the excessive fatigue that had dogged me for the past year.

"Are you tired, or are you weak? There is a difference."

Yes, there was. My lower limbs were fatigued; the upper limbs seemed weak. I gave him examples of what I meant. "And there's pain, too, particularly in my knee."

"Well, then, that is not myasthenia. Myasthenia is painless."

I didn't know about that, but certainly what I had was not painless. I told him about my sight, trying to make a clear-cut distinction between double and patchy vision. He listened to it all carefully and hardly interrupted. He asked about the incidence of illness in my past, but put no specific questions.

"Come on, let's have a look at you."

I undressed and sat on the edge of the couch. He stood in front of me, hands crossed, and studied my eyes. He took my hands, pulled my arms toward him and then slightly upwards.

"The right side of your trunk is smaller than the left."

"Yes. It's difficult to get clothes with a good fit."

"Stand up."

He extended the index finger of his right hand horizontally and raised it to the level of my eyes. I followed it with my eyes, up and down, up and down. He pointed his finger toward the ceiling, then moved it to my left. Facing forwards, I followed its movement with my eyes.

"Can you still see it?"

"Yes." It stopped.

"Tell me if anything happens."

"It's vee-ing. Now it's double. Now the images have moved away from each other."

"Cover your right eye. Has one disappeared?"

"Yes, the one nearest to me."

"Now cover your left eye."

"The one nearest the wall has gone."

He moved his finger to an equivalent position on my right. There was no trace of a second finger.

"The right eye cuts out. That *is* a myasthenic reaction."

I lifted myself onto the couch again and he examined each eye in turn. I was told to touch my nose and his finger alternately, first with the right index finger and then with the left. He moved his finger around, but I had no difficulty with the exercise, nor in finding my nose with either finger while my eyes were shut. There was no hand tremor then, or when I stretched my arms out forwards.

He took a pin and pressed it gently on the crown of my head. "Feel anything?"

"Yes."

He moved the pin down the side of my head, neck and upper

arms. Yes, I could feel it. But something in my demeanour, or the intonation of my voice, stopped him. He put both hands on the couch to my left and leaned on them.

"What can you feel? Pricks or pressure?"

"Well, I can feel it, but it doesn't prick."

"Look here, let's get down to first principles. A pin pricks or else it is not a pin. Got it? O.K. Let's start again." I did not feel a prick on any area - left or right - of my head, shoulders, arms or chest.

"Lie down." I felt a series of light indentations on the skin of my stomach, shins, upper insteps and the soles of my feet. The upper thighs were the areas of least sensitivity.

"Turn over." He started at the top and worked downwards again. Below the buttocks to approximately the knee I felt a pattern of definite sharp pricks.

"There's some sacral sparing, that's all."

The sensory loss which Green was exploring (and of which I had been largely unaware) is due to the compression of certain spinal nerves. However, sensation is often unimpaired over those areas which are supplied by the sacral segments of the spinal cord, and this is referred to as sacral sparing.

Green leaned against the door frame. "Your bath water - do you like it hot?"

"Um, very."

"How hot is very?"

"Well, my husband hates using the bathroom after me because it's like a sauna. My drinks, too, are either freezing cold or boiling hot. I take tea and coffee black and it has to come straight from the kettle. I don't taste much either - without chillis or loads of pepper or something, food isn't worth eating."

Green moved over to his table, picked up a tissue and brushed my right leg with it. "I can only just feel that." He exchanged it for cotton wool. "That's better."

He flourished the pin at me. "I'm telling you right now that you haven't got myasthenia."

While I tried to work that one out, he moved my big toes up and down. I had no difficulty in identifying their position. He elicited the usual reflexes, which seemed normal. The ankle reflexes were not brisk, but they were present, and none of the others were exaggerated. He then tested the legs for any signs of weakness; he found none, he said.

Green wrapped the steely-grey blood-pressure sleeve around my upper arm and inflated it. He whistled softly. "It's high."

"Oh? How high?"

"170. It could get you into trouble. I'll make arrangements for you to see a specialist physician."

His thoroughness, and the careful attention he seemed to pay to detail, impressed me.

"All right, get dressed and let's see if we can make anything of it."

I walked up to his desk, struggling with the buckle of my belt. He continued writing for a few seconds and then came around and sat next to me.

"Sit down. Do you know any anatomy?"

"A little."

He sketched the lower portion of the brain and the cervical spine. He added what he called a "horn" protruding from the cerebellum – the more usual term is "tonsil". He crooked the index finger of his right hand. "This is known as an Arnold-Chiari malformation." He explained that this is a lesion of the hindbrain, characterised by the downward displacement of the cerebellum and medulla through the foramen magnum into the cervical spinal canal. "That's your problem; you have a Chiari."

I looked at him. He was very alert, the arch-type of invincible certainty, and he issued his pronouncement with the unwavering ring of unassailable confidence.

And so, on 20th December, 1974, Bruce Green decided, after a conscientious medical examination lasting approximately three-quarters of an hour, that I had a congenital anomaly of the hindbrain and that this was responsible for fatigue and pain in my right leg, made walking a grave effort, and instigated attacks of double and patchy vision; it was also responsible for weakness and trembling in the right and – less frequently – the left arm and trunk, as well as the almost total loss of sensitivity over my entire body. I had not told him about the fits, now five in number, because I thought they would disappear as they had before.

Dr. Green may have made his pronouncement with unalloyed confidence, but he struck a discordant note in that moment that quivered in the air for many months to come, growing louder and louder until it reached an ear-splitting crescendo. Nevertheless, he never changed the orchestration, although he did add a variation, which he played with concentration, if not talent. Or maybe that was his little scherzo, and I just lack a sense of humour.

I studied the man guardedly. He was dealing with the most complex matter on earth, which yields the elusive secrets of its labyrinthine functioning in health and in sickness only very reluctantly, if at all. I had tried to avoid inept fumbling, but rash synthetic exuberance could be equally dangerous, and here he was, jumping in boots and all. Was he mad? Was he arrogant? Or was he, perhaps, right?

Green is a pleasant man with an easy manner, capable of warmth and utterly devoid of ersatz charm. Moreover, I do not think one needs to be a dedicated student of cognitive psychology to recognise that he is scarcely an indifferent neurologist. I was not in possession of facts on which to base a judgment either of the relative balance of his mind, or of the validity of his diagnosis. But at least he did not come across as arrogant; it was not so much a question of insolent pride as imprudent certitude, less haughty self-importance than importunate self-assurance. And if he was not indubitably perspicacious, neither was he obtuse.

Much later I came to the conclusion that these ego-trips must be the essential lubricant in his psychic equipment. At that moment I was faced with the question: should I stay or should I go? In the end intellectual curiosity won the day. If he was right, I had a great deal more to learn about psychomotor disturbance than I had ever imagined, and it would be a lesson that might prove salutary in my work with young children.

"I want you to have your skull and neck X-rayed, and a full battery of blood tests taken – you know, sugar, potassium, blood counts, the lot."

I looked askance at him, waiting for him to bring up the subject of the high blood pressure, but he did not. I decided to leave it for the time being.

My friend Jill was in the waiting room, head back against the wall above the seat, eyes closed. She opened them and glanced at me sharply. I looked back unsmilingly and we left the rooms in silence.

"Well?"

I did not answer. She gave another verbal prod and I told her in detail what had taken place. Her eyes – dark, stony – never left my face. Jill, herself the wife of a specialist, is highly qualified in neuropsychology and pharmacology; her husband once remarked, jokingly, that she knew more about the latter than he did.

"The man is mad," she said in a dull, flat tone.

"I think he was precipitous." I felt uncomfortable; I do not like smart alecks, and it seemed to me that he came close to being one. But I made up my mind there and then that if I was going to continue to consult him, and there did not seem to be a good alternative, I would have to banish or at least subdue my doubts; I was not going to start acting as my own diagnostician.

4

Jill was again with me when on 8th January, 1975, I went for the exclusion tests for myasthenia. Electromyography is a bioelectric recording technique similar in principle to the EEG and ECG. In this case electric charges are recorded from a muscle stimulated by a small electrode inserted into the fleshy pad at the base of the thumb. The chains of oscillations generated by the muscular activity appear in emerald on a TV-like screen that is appropriately calibrated. Green indicated the cut-off point of the oscillations in a normal polygraph, and on the first try they remained within this limit.

"Hey, wait a minute, they're going over."

Green repeated the tests several times, but the results were so equivocal that he counted them as negative. Had I been recording them under experimental conditions, I would have done the same. He tried Tensilon, injecting it into my right arm. He moved the index finger of his left hand to the left of my eyes.

"It's vee-ing. There are two. They've moved apart."

His finger remained quite still. "Any change?"

"No."

"Sure?"

"Yes."

He waited a few seconds, keeping his finger steady. "Now?"

"No." He had two fingers, and that was that.

"Well, that certainly isn't a positive reaction." I slipped off the couch. "Look, nothing is going to convince me that you have myasthenia, but I'll put you on a course of Mestinon."

Mestinon has certain chemical properties that make it possible to diagnose fairly accurately whether a patient has myasthenia gravis or not. Somebody who has this disease shows a favourable response to the drug that is generally dramatic and sustained.

"Nothing on the X-rays?" I queried.

"No." I was amused by his faint air of pugnacity. There is something of the Churchillian bulldog about Green.

"Blood tests?"

"No." He averted his eyes, turned his back and wrote out a script. "See me in a fortnight."

Every day I took the prescribed three Mestinons, which come only in a strength of 60 mg. I did feel better, less lethargic, and in particular less weak in the shoulder and neck area. However, my walking did not improve, the cramps became more severe and so did the pain in the knee.

I saw Green again on 22nd January.

"I feel better. I think the Mestinon has helped."

"You shouldn't feel better on Mestinon, because you have not got myasthenia."

I laughed. I was not going to argue to the contrary; after all, the polygraph was normal and the results of the second Tensilon test were negative. However, I did think that the two doctors had been looking for different signs. "O.K. But I still feel that the Mestinon helps."

"Psychologically, perhaps."

"If that's what you think, put me onto placebos as well." A pill or potion which is a placebo is inert, and has no active pharmacologic ingredient. But its psychologic effect can be marked, and so it is offered as "something to please the patient".

I did not know how the very distinctive taste of Mestinon could be simulated so that the placebo could not be distinguished on that basis, but it seemed to be a good way of keeping Green in touch with neurologic reality. After all, it is not impossible for general or symptomatic myasthenia to respond to Mestinon, although the reaction is rarely dramatic and often ceases within a few weeks. Certainly, there appeared to be no lasting effects so far as I was concerned.

"I might just do that, but let's have a look at you meantime."

I undressed and sat on the couch; he faced me exactly as before. His eyes narrowed a little as he stared intently at mine.

"The left pupil is much bigger than the other. When did that happen?"

"Oh, I noticed it for the first time about ten months ago."

"Nonsense. It wasn't like that before; I'm sure, because it's the sort of thing I watch out for."

I stared at him in astonishment. I thought he had looked at me carefully on the first occasion. "My eyes haven't been normal for a long time; that is precisely the reason I am here. The left pupil is always dilated, sometimes more so than others, and the right one is always constricted. And the ptosis also varies quite a bit - it can be dreadful. How is it now?"

"It's certainly there."

I went up to the mirror above the handbasin. "It's fine today."

Green proceeded with the examination. He could not elicit double vision, although he held his finger stationary at the usual distance from the left side of my face for several minutes.

"I'm prepared to stand here for as long as it takes."

"Well, you can forget about your dinner then - the finger isn't budging."

I thought that the insensitivity to the pin pricks had increased; there was still sacral sparing, but the pin had lost some of its potency in this region. When Green began visually to compare the one leg with the other, I complained, loud and clear, about my difficulties with the right one. He examined it scrupulously; there was no local pain and he denied that there was any weakness.

"Look, I think I ought to do a myelogram. If nothing shows up, we'll just have to sit tight."

As he got to the door I stopped him.

"You're sure about the myasthenia?"

"*Yes.*"

"No myasthenia?"

"Absolutely *no* myasthenia."

"Well, what's the matter with my eyes? Why the ptosis?"

"You've got a Horner's syndrome there." This is recognised by a slight ptosis (which is not, strictly speaking, a "lazy eyelid", though one often hears it referred to as such), as well as contraction of the pupil of the eye on the affected side. That side of the face may also become flushed, and mine did, many times. But as I did not then see any connection, and because it seemed a rather paltry thing to mention, I did not.

"Oh, and where does a Horner's, whatever that is, come from?"

36

He gave a karate-like chop at the side of his neck with the inner edge of his right hand. "It's due to the Chiari."

5

On 28th January I was admitted to Lords Nursing Home for the myelogram. This involves introducing a radio-opaque iodised fluid, in this case Myodil, into the spinal cord by means of a lumbar puncture. Following the injection, the patient is safely secured on a tilting table under an X-ray screen. X-rays are taken at appropriate levels as the Myodil flows along the spine towards the head. The iodised oil acts as a dye, so that abnormalities can be more easily detected.

I expected an ordeal, but was pleasantly surprised. The procedure is quite painless; the only discomfort was caused by the gravity-defying upside-down position that was necessary to encourage the movement of the Myodil towards the head, to where a lesion near the foramen magnum was suspected. It was all over very quickly and I was returned to my bed with strict instructions from Green not to move for the next twelve hours if I wanted to avoid a post-lumbar-puncture headache.

At about 5 p.m. that evening a very bad bout of leg spasms and cramp in the toes began, probably triggered by the Myodil. I gripped the head rail with both hands and felt the sweat beading my face. I hung on for twenty minutes before I rang for the sister. Fifteen minutes later she came in.

"Green's here now, I'll get him." She returned with a syringe.

"What's that?"

"Valium."

"I want Green, not Valium."

"No, look, let me give you this. It will help that leg – it's a muscle relaxant."

"Not until Green has seen my leg, thanks."

"It's nothing to worry about, just a reaction to the myelogram."

"Yeah, maybe. But I go through this every morning of my life, Myodil or no Myodil. It's slightly more severe now, but it's identical in every other way. I want Green to see it."

He came in and watched in silence as the leg convulsed. "You know those horns I told you about?" He crooked that index finger. "You've got one."

I could not mistake the triumphant look on his face. So he *was* right. If I had not *been* on my back, I would have *fallen* on it, and I told him so. He looked like the proverbial Cheshire cat, although the grin was confined to his eyes.

"So that *is* what my problem is?"

"Yes. I am going to ask Mr. Aschen to look at you. He knows much more about Chiaris than I do. But I don't think he'll operate. I would be prepared to accept that, the lesion is very mild. I'm leaving the Myodil in; he may want to rescreen you."

So it wasn't quite a Chiari; only a chiari. My mind ticked over. The anomaly was minor; its manifestations were not.

I began to push the diagnosis around mentally. I twisted this way and that, balking at every turn. After fifteen years of intensive study of man's mind in both good functioning and bad, my memory store of neuropsychological information suddenly stalled. The link between my pathology and a Chiari (and certainly a chiari) would not gel. I gave a wry shrug – I must have read all the wrong books.

As far as the myelogram was concerned, I was apparently one of the lucky ones. As Green said later, I didn't turn a hair; there was no reaction whatever to the procedure, apart from a slight dizziness when I left the bed for the first time the following afternoon.

The leg spasms had undoubtedly become worse during the evening and night following the injection of the Myodil. I overheard Green inform the sister when they left my ward that the dye would have to be removed in the morning. From the brief monologue that drifted in from the corridor I gleaned that Green was rather reluctant to do this, because it was unlikely that Aschen would see me immediately. He was very busy, too.

Aschen came in on the second day after the myelogram. He went over more or less the same ground Green had covered on his first examination. He seemed surprised at the extent of the loss of sensitivity to pin pricks.

"This sort of cloak effect generally does not extend much below mid-trunk." He repeated the test and shook his head, plainly puzzled. But he was no more taken aback than Green had been when he first made this discovery.

Aschen turned his attention to my eyes. "Why do you keep tilting your head to the right?"

"I can't see clearly unless I do."

He picked up a magazine. "Read this." I did so, easily. "You are still tilting your head. Keep it straight. Any difference?"

"Yes, a bit. The ink is less bright in some parts than in others."

"That will do. Let's see what your walking is like."

I walked across the room, returned heel-to-toe, heel-to-toe. I stood on one leg and then the other, eyes open, eyes shut. I did not do very well. I told him that in this respect there had not been much change over many years: I had been a clumsy, badly co-ordinated child. My current concern was the inability to walk any distance, and the constant giving at the knee and the leg spasms and pain.

"Mrs. Birrer, I think you have a very mild Chiari, but I would be most unwilling indeed, in fact I would not be prepared at all, to do anything about it."

"You mean, anything surgical?"

"Yes."

"*I* wouldn't contemplate surgery at this time. Anyway, what chance is there that surgery would fix it?"

He shrugged. "Our work on the Chiari is only about ten years old. Every case is idiosyncratic."

"What happens to a Chiari? Does it get worse?"

"In my experience, it fluctuates."

When Green came in the next morning to discharge me, I asked him the same question.

"In my experience, it throws up symptoms. The equivocal ones are the difficult ones."

I did not like it one bit. A lesion so capricious that its very existence seemed uncertain, with all-embracing consequences, sounded more like an alchemist's conundrum than a serious medical explanation of the queer quotidian events of the past year. Nor was it a happy augury.

"You can go home now."

"Not so fast. What are you going to do about my leg?"

"I can't do anything about it. It's a Chiari leg."

"You mean, it's a live-with-it leg?"

"Yes."

We stared at each other for a long moment. "There must be *something* you can do about the spasms."

He looked wary. "Try Benadryl, two tablespoons in the evening.

See me in a fortnight."

Benadryl is usually given for an allergic condition, particularly hay fever. I picked up the script when I left the nursing home with the Myodil still in my spine.

I rushed to the phone as soon as I arrived home. I wanted to make sure that my students did not read the wrong books, too.

"Mr. Aschen, Mrs. Birrer speaking. This thing that I've got, this Chiari. It's most interesting but quite perplexing, really. Dr. Green says you know all there is to know about it. I wonder if you would give an informal talk to some members of our staff and a group of students on the subject. As psychologists, they could derive a lot of benefit from it."

He declined, very politely. He did not think that enough was known about the Chiari to be able to relate it reliably to psychological functioning.

6

I had not had an attack of double vision since I began taking Mestinon. However, the frequency of the fits increased; in a way, they seemed to have taken the place of the double vision. Now, when I began to feel ill, I anticipated a fit. According to those who saw them, these too had a typical pattern: head snapping backwards, eyes open, pronounced stiffening of limbs, crying out and falling unless held. Following a short period of thrashing and straining strongly to the right, I would remain quiet but unconscious for more or less twenty minutes, and afterwards remember nothing except the tell-tale preliminaries. As in the case of the spells of double vision, I had to go to sleep immediately, although this was less of an inconvenience, since the fits rarely occurred before late afternoon.

I was driving along Louis Botha Avenue one morning in the first week of February when the area over my left ribs began to feel numb. By the time I reached Corlett Drive about ten minutes later, it had stiffened; I lowered my left shoulder and leaned sideways, pushing my waist toward the right in an effort to slacken the tautening skin. My left arm was not affected at all, but by now I was so uncomfortable that I stopped the car. I looked uneasily at the thin black body shirt stretched tightly over my trunk and stomach. A strip about 5 cm in width, slightly to the left of the mid-line, extending from breast to navel, corded and arched up. It began to pulsate regularly and strongly, causing acute discomfort. It did not last long and I went on my way. However, it happened again that evening while I was sitting in the bath, legs stretched out. It recurred six or seven times more under these circumstances. I decided it probably had something to do with the position of my legs.

It was about this time that I first experienced some difficulty with my speech. I knew what it was that I wanted to say, the words were on the tip of my tongue, but its previous almost involuntary activity now required conscious effort. I would struggle for a while, mumbling and stumbling, but I did manage to get it all out after a minute or so, generally with undue emphasis. Rarely a day passed without a small incident of this nature. I found the lapses so distressing that I spoke about them constantly to Jill.

I arrived ten minutes early for my third visit to Green on 14th February. With my right hand on the steering wheel I turned towards the back seat for my book. Almost immediately the band of skin on the left roped up and began to throb painfully. I sat and watched it for a full five minutes, wondering all the time whether I should go up to the surgery and let Green see it. I decided against disturbing him; I did, after all, have a tongue, even if I had to work a bit harder now for its co-operation.

In fact, when I got into his consulting room I felt embarrassed about mentioning such an implausible development, but Green heard me out without interruption; I could see that the story was one of the most interesting I had told him.

"You won't find that in any of the books. But I have had a patient who had the identical thing. I thought this patient was mad until I saw it one day for myself, in the rooms. We are going to have to go up higher." He tapped his forehead with his index finger.

I told him about the fits, which had begun in September but were now increasing both in severity and frequency. I also told him that they did not bother me particularly, since there were always warning signals. I was beginning to realise that, apart from feeling ill just beforehand, I was particularly prone to falling and to crashing into things during the days immediately preceding an attack, again always on the right, so that abnormal bruising on both the right upper arm and leg were definite signals of an impending fit. I stressed as well my concern about the lapses of halting and indistinct speech.

On 17th February I went to a research institute for my first electroencephalogram. For an EEG, electrodes are attached to the skull with a jelly that spells disaster to any hair style. A graphic record of the wavy changes in the electric activity of the brain is made under varying conditions: eyes open, eyes shut, over-breathing (or hyperventilation), flicker (or photic stimulation) from a light source that switches on and off at ever increasing rates. Children apparently often find this very soothing; it pushed me to the brink of unconsciousness.

"Tell them I'm looking for parasurgical lesions of the brain," Green had instructed me. Perhaps they knew what he meant, but I have never been able to find out.

It was an uncomfortable session. When I hyperventilated, as I was asked to do, the sole of my right foot roped out, becoming so stiff that I had to kick off the constricting shoe. It was the first time I remember having leg spasms during the day.

On 18th February a brain scan was taken. This is isotope encephalography. It works on the principle that a tumour (or other brain lesion) absorbs an excessive amount of a radioactive substance, enabling it to be detected radiographically. A positive finding is highly significant, but a negative one does not exclude the possibility of a tumour. Green's patient who had the spasms over her ribs was by this procedure found to have a large tumour. In my case the results were negative.

When I saw Green again on 3rd March the only new development was four ordinary faints. Twice I had fallen straight forward, eyes closed, onto the dinner table, and twice I had passed out briefly at the university.

"Forward faints are quite characteristic of a Chiari," Green said, mimicking the action of falling forward with his right hand.

"What about the fits?"

"There's something funny on the EEG."

"Funny?"

"Well, there's something in the temporal area. The institute wants to repeat the EEG in six weeks. I think you should. Meanwhile, I'll try you on an anti-convulsant. Let's see – Epanutin, I think. Take two a day."

42

A week later I reported by phone that my right leg was no longer convulsing, but that it had become spastic instead; nor was there any decrease in the number of fits.

"Step the Epanutin up to three a day."

I did so. At 100 mg a time, I was now every day taking 300 mg of the drug.

Within two weeks of starting the Epanutin I found that the spasms in my right leg had disappeared completely. I was overjoyed; I could thrash around in bed to my heart's content without any hint of a convulsion. But although the spasms in the leg were gone, the pain had not. The spasm on the left side of the trunk also did not recur, nor did the faints; the severity of the fits had lessened, although their frequency was unaffected.

However, it was obviously too much to expect that there would be no further complications. I had several hour-long sessions of complete hearing loss, when I watched the students in front of me open and shut their mouths like so many gulping goldfish. I can recall three such occasions, after which I only experienced partial loss, usually in the left ear. I phoned Green and he told me to drop into his rooms on the way home from work.

He examined my leg. "Show me just where the pain is." I pointed. "But you've never had pain there before."

I could not believe my ears. "Of course I have, but now the concomitant spasms have gone."

"You are talking yourself into a specialist physician."

"Don't be silly."

"No, really, you may have a clot there. You should have it checked."

I had my own ideas about the existence of a clot which did not have much to do with my right leg. "I'll go and have a chat to my husband's G.P."

I knew that he had discussed the case with Green on one occasion, when Bill had seen him about a problem of his own. This would obviate my having to go over the whole long, dreary story again.

"Just check my blood pressure, will you?" He did so.

"What is it?"

"170," he replied, tersely.

Green wrote a short note and I went immediately to Charles Meter, with whom both Bill and I had a very warm relationship.

"Charles, what is my blood pressure?"

He encased my upper arm in the sleeve. "140."

"Are you sure?"

He repeated the exercise, twice more. "Sure I'm sure. Why?"

"According to Green, it's 170. Didn't he mention it?"

"No." Meter chuckled. "Funny thing, he always gets a high reading. I think patients are just plain scared of neurologists."

I plucked at the sheet. I wasn't having much fun, but I wasn't afraid, either - not of doctors, anyway.

"Please see if there is any wax in my ears. I'm not hearing so well."

"Not a thing there."

I told him about the pain in my leg. He checked the blood pressure in both legs, which was identical, and also did an ECG, which is a bioelectric technique of recording the spreading electric potentials that accompany the cycle of the heart beat. "Absolutely normal."

He leaned against the couch, arms folded, and studied my eyes. I knew that the ptosis was very pronounced and the left pupil almost fully dilated. "How much Mestinon are you taking?"

"None."

"Why ever not?"

"Because I haven't got myasthenia."

"Who says so?"

"The electromyograph and the Tensilon say so."

"Rubbish. It's only a machine, and machines can make mistakes."

"Yes, I know. And so does Green. That's why he tried the Mestinon."

"What does he think about the eye?"

"Apparently it's a Horner's, due to the Chiari."

"Who says you've got a Chiari?"

"The X-ray says so, and Green says so, and Aschen thinks so - at least, that's what I think he thinks."

"I don't believe it. It's only an X-ray. X-rays are a notorious source of defective diagnoses."

"Just wait a bit - are you saying that I *have* got myasthenia, although according to Green the clinical picture contradicts this, and the tests are negative, and that I do *not* have a Chiari, although the X-ray as well as a neurologist and neurosurgeon are of the opinion that I do?"

He did not reply. "Tell me, Charles, if I had a temperature of 40, would you be worried?"

"Well, yes, if you had a high temperature, of course I'd be worried."

"Why? It's only a thermometer?"

We stared at each other. "Do you think the hearing loss could be due to the Epanutin?" I asked. "The two do coincide."

He reached for the faithful Mims, the pharmacological what's what.

"It doesn't say so. What are you taking Epanutin for?"

"A temporal focus - I think." According to the EEG report, whatever dysfunction there was, was probably related to the temporal area of the brain.

"Look, Cynthia, I'm telling you something - your doctors are making you sick."

Well, that was a fact, but I did not intend to pursue the subject.

"Charles, my leg is giving me a lot of trouble. Can't you do anything? Green reckons it's a Chiari leg, but Epanutin has suppressed the spasms - surely there is something that will help for the pain? Honestly, I don't know how you chaps make it out of medical school."

"Yes, I'm sure we can do something about that." He scribbled on his pad and handed the page to me. I glanced down at it.

"Good God, this is for Serepax, tranquillisers. A few weeks ago Green prescribed Benadryl for the same thing. I'm not mad, you know - the pain's in my leg, not my head."

He smiled soothingly. "Give it a go for three weeks - you'll feel much better - and keep on with the Mestinon."

I walked out. Well, I would not repeat *that* caper again.

7

Green had the results of the second EEG when I saw him on 8th April. The picture had not changed, and another reading in six weeks was advised. I told him bitterly that I now had a lot of pain in the right leg, and that walking was not easy.

"Patients with a Chiari often get pains down the legs." He ran both hands down one of his own.

"It's only the right leg. Are you quite sure about that wretched Chiari?"

"It's there all right."

"I just don't know. I'm getting so damned fatigued again, it's difficult to get around."

"I think it's neurasthenia."

"Do you mean a *neurotic* fatigue?"

"Yes."

"Psychosomatic?"

"Yes."

I hooted. "My friend, in this case neurasthenia, if you define it like that, is as mythical as you claim myasthenia to be."

"I don't know – you've had problems."

I looked at him sharply. What on earth was he referring to? He noticed my stupefaction.

"I mean, you have *got* problems."

"Yes, and I suppose they must be creating some anxiety – it would be extraordinary if they were not. But there's a great deal more to it than that."

Since man is a thinking being, psychological phenomena are involved in any disease, even if only in the form of anxiety or despair. But labelling a patient neurasthenic or neurotic because these factors undeniably play a part in pathology seems to me to be a very queer ploy indeed. Way out, in fact. Actually, among doctors, Green is the worst psychologist I have come across in my various experiences as a patient. And in this particular instance he was doubly out of order because it was one of his own breed, the great French neurologist Pierre Janet, who first showed that it is quite worthless to define the neuroses in terms of the intervention of psychologic phenomena.

"How much Mestinon are you taking?"

"I stopped them. You're so certain about the myasthenia there doesn't seem much point in taking the pills."

"No, no, go back to them. You said you felt better on them. Try them again. I'm a firm believer in clinical medicine," he said with conviction. Or at least, he seemed convinced. I never thought that soon a dozen dawns would come when I would wonder what it was that prevented him from practising what he believed.

I had my third EEG on 3rd May. I phoned Green for the results, which he said were unchanged. Actually, there was some deterioration. I had felt much the same during the preceding six weeks, but now events took a steep plunge downward. The fits were occurring almost daily and apparently were often quite violent. But other things were happening too.

One Sunday morning in April I propped myself up in bed and, with breakfast next to me, read the national newspapers. I was thick-headed and uncomfortable in the stomach. I thought a splash of cold water might help. I twisted the taps and glanced in the mirror. A strangely lop-sided apparition was reflected back. I stared, mildly mystified. The *right* pupil was fully dilated and the *left* one constricted. By 11 a.m. I was feeling ghastly, but I knew, somehow, that it did not betoken an attack of double vision. I lay down, becoming more ill by the minute, aware of a rapid build-up of pressure in my head. I thought I could detect some activity, unusual movements within the head itself. What was quite definite, however, was the real fear that gripped my guts. Dear God, I was going to have a cerebral haemorrhage; please, please, let it be a big one, let it be final. I could not tolerate the thought of brain surgery, of comatose states, of an eternal vigil by the faithful over an inert, uncomprehending form, watching through days and weeks and months for the slightest indication of a return to consciousness. I had seen it happen to others; it could not happen to me.

I opened my mouth to scream, but no sound came. I strained and strained, but it was no use. My hands were wet and icy. The one thing I really did dread was going to happen, and I had to face it on my own. My head exploded and I lost consciousness.

When I came around my head was less tight, but within seconds there was a fresh upsurge and another shattering explosion, followed by a third.

It was after 1 p.m. before I felt myself again, a little dazed, but much better. It was the first of the head explosions; like the double vision and the fits, the attacks were always similar, their frequency increased rapidly and there was the same compulsion subsequently to sleep and sleep and sleep. I lost the initial paralytic fear when it seemed clear that there was not going to be a haemorrhage after all, but I was never able to call out or shout.

Another development during this period was lengthy chains of spasms that convulsed the shoulder and the right arm above the elbow. As the jerking became pronounced I would grip biceps and shoulder alternately, in an effort to suppress the insistent movement. Once, at a matinee performance, I spooned up an ice-cream during the interval and then had to spend a harrowing half-hour in the cloakroom trying to control the violent convulsions. On a few occasions the convulsions were preceded by twitching and pain on the right side of the face and trembling in the hand.

I walked into Green's room again on 7th July. He had the report of the fourth EEG of 25th June in his hand. He passed it to me over the desk. There had been a marked deterioration.

"What am I going to do with you?"

"I don't know; but I do know that things are going downhill - fast." I went over it all in detail. He watched me quietly. "Some things seem to be so wrong, and yet others are still going well - my writing, for example."

There was a marked silence. "I am quite prepared to accept that an EEG is only a piece of paper until I hear the kinds of things you're saying. Then I get cold feet. I must do an angiogram." In this procedure a dye is injected into the left carotid artery in the neck to facilitate X-raying the arterial system in the head.

I hesitated. There was something on my mind, but I could not bring myself to say it. "You think an angiogram is necessary?"

"The EEG report indicates that it is, and so does your story. Frankly, I'm chicken. Go and get undressed."

As usual I sat on the couch. He stared at me and gave an involuntary start. "I have never seen your ptosis like that. It is awful."

"Yes. Sometimes I have the greatest difficulty in keeping the eye open at all."

Green always took pains with his examinations, but this time he was back-checking. Everything was much as before - no double vision, same extent of insensitivity to pin pricks - until he started on the reflexes. There was no response from either ankle. He tapped the knee, eliciting a series of rapid and exaggerated contractions. He tried again, with the same result, and then again.

"Shit." That was my sentiment, too. Seconds later I felt the oncoming rush of a head explosion. The upper portion of the right arm and shoulder began to convulse violently. I twisted onto my right, lifting my left side off the couch. I leant heavily on the upper right arm. The shoulder shuddered and writhed. I leaned harder, feeling the panic rising. I also felt a bit sick. Green's astounded eyes were glued to my arm.

"It's your *shoulder*," he exclaimed, unable to refrain from stating the obvious.

"I get . . ." I tried to force out a sentence, but I could only make the harsh, rasping sound that was characteristic of these attacks and that always prevented me from calling for help. I made another effort.

"Don't talk while it's happening."

I let the avalanche take its course. My head exploded twice before the disturbance subsided. I asked for a drink of water. Green was grave, brooding.

"I don't know what that is." He was almost inaudible.

He rang for a syringe. "I'm going to try Tensilon again."

His gaze never left my right eye when he had given the injection. "Definitely no reaction."

He helped me off the couch. We stood facing each other. "I must do the angiogram." He ran his finger down my neck. "I expect it to be negative," he said firmly. But he was shaken, and it was not at all clear that he really did.

I went out to his desk and sat down. He turned to his phone. "Now, about that angiogram. . . ."

"No, no angiogram."

There was no doubt that further neurologic investigation was clearly indicated. But an angiogram is used to detect abnormal vascularity, for example, in an aneurysm, or the displacement of the cerebral arteries by a tumour. I could not see that my problems were necessarily being caused by either. Eventually, I supposed, the possibility of both had to be excluded, but right now I thought Green ought to review the whole case with a colleague, just to make sure he was not barking up the wrong tree, diagnostically speaking. There *are* other things besides aneurysms and brain tumours that can affect the nervous system in strange ways. I could not shake off the vague feeling that something was being overlooked.

Green fingered the receiver. "You don't have to have it if you don't want it." His forehead furrowed. "But you *must*. What are you going to do if that happens in a lecture?"

"It has. What are you going to do if the angiogram shows nothing?"

"I am going to push pills."

"Drug therapy?"

"Drug therapy," he affirmed, nodding his head.
I nodded too, wordlessly. I had to leave it to him.

8

The psychologically most stressful period during the progressive capitulation of my body to disease started towards the end of March 1975. I had begun to feel desperately ill. The experience was not entirely novel; the bouts of double vision and fits had always been heralded by an acute physical unease, but now this was magnified a thousand-fold. Green wanted to know exactly what I meant when I said I felt ill, and I was rendered helpless and frustrated by his probings, floundering in a inchoate welter.

"Headache?"

"No."

"Nausea?"

"No."

"Pain?"

"No."

"Well, what then?"

"Peculiar, just peculiar."

From the look on his face, he obviously thought me so too. But it was impossible to put the sensation into words. When I tried they echoed as hollowly as the strained and stilted vocabulary the English language offers to lovers, and I could not rescue the rhetoric from its shackles as a Michener might do, falling back on some graphic and picturesque argot.

Over twenty years I have developed a good sense of the functioning of my own body. Among other things, I am aware of when I begin to ovulate, even though my cycle is irregular, and it is easy to describe the process in such terms as heaviness, or fullness, or distension, or whatever the immediate experience is. But in this situation there were no really appropriate linguistic labels. Somewhere, deep inside, I was undergoing destruction by some form of physiological pollution, much as the mind might disintegrate under the impact of the subtle and insidious persuasion of the Chinese water treatment. There was a strong feeling of dissolution, of decomposition, a loss of the definition of internal boundaries, a gradual but resolute slak-ing of tissue rendering the body anomalous, and it was as if the cumulative effects were being swept through every vessel by the blood, suffocating vitality. It was a rapacious invasion of the vital principle that destroyed its power to quicken; it would not be repuls-ed, and it made me feel very sick indeed.

After the worst attack I suffered during the period of head explo-sions, I stood staring out of my bedroom window at the cascading grace of the weeping willow, sweeping and sinuous in the afternoon balm against the white garden wall. I no longer felt ill, but in my heart of hearts I knew that all the king's horses and all the king's men were not going to be able to put together the pieces inside me again. I understood then, in an idiosyncratic way, the incorporeal predator that had been my constant companion for at least the pre-ceding twenty-one months. It was my first real grasp of the Kafkaes-que dimensions of my condition, and while I never dwelt on it, it prepared me for the unvarnished truth when I was forced to face it. It also enabled me to take the first steps towards my own emotional rehabilitation. What I had lost on the swings I gained on the round-abouts.

I mentioned the experience to Jill on the Thursday before the an-giogram. We were sipping tea from heavy brown pottery mugs in the cosiness of the playroom in her home. Preoccupied, I watched two-year-old Sally covering her doll with a gaily crocheted blanket and then uncovering it, repeating her actions again and yet again.

"You should have had the angio on Tuesday – it was a mistake to wait a week."

"I suppose so. But I'm not worried about that any more. I really don't think there's anything there. It's something else, something de-generative . . ."

We looked at each other, me and this woman with her uncanny ability to fathom the tortuous convolutions of the human mind. The silence seemed to press down on us. The clock struck two. We picked up our mugs and talked of other things.

9

After rushing to tie up some of those interminable loose ends I was admitted into the nursing home around 11.30 a.m. on 15th July. At 1 p.m., knotted into the appropriate off-white, starched hospital gown, stripped of jewels and devoid of make-up – I chewed my lipstick off, but a nurse took care of the nail polish with swatches of cotton wool saturated in acetone – I was given an injection that was supposed to make me drowsy, but which had no effect. I intended to ward off oblivion until I had heard the results of the angiogram.

The procedure was painless and quick, so that it was not long before Green hissed into my ear:

"There is nothing in your kop. Give thanks."

I took that to mean that there was nothing inside my head that should not be there. And, God, I was grateful and told Him so.

I awoke twice during the afternoon, the first time to tell my parents and Jill the good news and later, when Green popped in. I did not have a brain tumour, and he was genuinely delighted with the discovery.

"While you're here I'll get Mr. Aschen to check you over."

"But is it necessary? I'm not going to have an operation."

"No. But he might just as well see you while you're here."

During his regular visit the following morning I told Green that since he insisted I see Mr. Aschen, I would again raise the question of my right leg with him.

"I haven't complained about it much recently. If it is a Chiari leg, as you insist, I suppose I do have to live with it, but the pain is about forty per cent worse."

He circled my chair, right arm akimbo, a characteristic pose. "Well, how bad is it?"

"Pretty bad. But I can cope, as long as it doesn't get any worse."

"But can you? Maybe I should do some arm twisting – your's and Asch's. I don't want to, though. I'm a pacifist."

"No, definitely, no. I think surgery is premature. I'd rather go on until, say, December; see how things develop. But if I really can't manage, I'll come to you."

He dropped his arm, nodded, turned and walked away.

I watched his receding back. Having a modicum of knowledge of the complexity of the nervous system, I was going to make haste slowly. Green had persuaded me – albeit not completely – that the pain in my leg, as well as the difficulty I had walking, were due to that ephemeral Chiari; and that *if* the faints and fits were not, at least they would be controlled by Pushing Pills. But I never really understood how a Chiari – or a temporal lesion, for that matter – could account for the spells of double vision and the blurred sight that had persisted for twelve months. And *that,* after all, was where it had all begun.

Could it be that a Chiari – at least the now-you-see-it-now-you-don't variety – was just a dilettante, a puckish simulator? Maybe then – an outside chance I brushed aside the moment it entered my mind – the matter was not so neatly wrapped up, after all. I did not find the prospect particularly alarming. I had been told, by men whose judgment I thought could be trusted, that Green was a Brilliant Neurologist, and the odd disquieting conjectures of a layman provided me with no valid grounds to question their opinion. I was quite confident that, regardless of what lay ahead, Green would see me safely through the woods. What is more, he knew perfectly well that I trusted him to do so, because I had written to him to that effect. I mean, if you hand out the brickbats, you should also be willing to bestow the accolades.

At 6 p.m. that day Green discharged me from the nursing home. He increased the Tegretol that he had started me on the week previously to three per day to control my Queer Fits. Green told me that Tegretol, an anti-convulsant, was his choice of drug because "there is temporal lobe involvement". In addition to the Epanutin, I was now swallowing 600 mg of Tegretol every day.

"Phone me in four weeks. Let me know how it's going."

I looked at Green quizzically. It was *excessively* difficult to get him on the telephone – *why* is the 64 000 rand question. Maybe the women who got into such a leggy tangle in reception had been instructed to block calls whenever the temperature in the surgery rose. Or perhaps they personally assumed the awesome responsibility of deciding who should, and who should not, speak to the doctor, just for fun. Phoney fun, to lighten the daily grind. Or maybe Green simply had an aversion to speaking to patients on the phone, because there were many times when he must simply have refused to take a call. What else does the short delay sandwiched between the tell-tale clicks of an internal connection mean? There were also times when Green gave his receptionist an answer to pass on, and the interchange between the two, while she tried to get it all straight, was clearly audible at the other end of the line. It would have made no difference to Green to say the same thing into a mouthpiece, but it would have made a considerable difference to the patient: some people like their messages first-hand, straight from the oracle himself. Whatever the reason, however, Green rarely took calls over the telephone - from me, at least - and the responsibility for his failure to do so rests squarely on his sturdy shoulders.

If I had known then that in the course of the next few months he would on ten occasions refuse to speak to me, and on four to my husband, whose distress at my imminent collapse knew no bounds, I would have thrashed the matter out right then and there. As it was, I had in the past always managed to get through to him eventually, and I naïvely expected that I would do so again whenever it was really necessary in the future, even if it was an exasperating and time-consuming business. *Of course* I would phone him in four weeks' time.

I wafted out of the nursing home on a pink cloud. Mr. Aschen considered that the Chiari had fluctuated and that it was less of a problem now than it had been in January, and it was mild then. Also, I definitely did not have myasthenia; an injection into the right arm of a heavy dose of curare, which causes paralysis in a myasthenic, had induced nothing more than a few spots before the eyes. Obviously there was only one way to go, and that was up. The family toasted the turn of the tide in champagne and we set our faces towards a rosy tomorrow. At 7.30 a.m. on Thursday, 17th July, I slipped into my office at the university to pick up the threads.

10

Exactly seven days after my discharge from the nursing home I attended a meeting in Pretoria and returned in the late afternoon. Home was still some way ahead when suddenly I was unable to depress the accelerator. I could feel neither the right leg nor the right foot and I certainly had no control whatever over either. I drew off the motor-way onto the grassy bank to await the return of some feeling in that offending member. However, after thirty minutes it remained as recalcitrant as before. I jogged the driver's seat forward as far as the steering wheel would allow and started slowly homeward, using my left leg dangerously in a dual capacity.

The rest of the journey was nightmarish; when it was over I dragged myself out of the car, landing with a wobble on my left leg. The right leg was still unwilling to respond at all, so I made unsteadily for the safety of my bed.

The unpleasant tingling in the right foot which woke me the following morning continued throughout that day and the next, subsiding a little toward the end of the third day. I was limping badly and flights of stairs became as formidable as Everest. Time and time again both ankle and knee gave way and I would stumble. I fell on several occasions. I began deliberately, and very successfully, to throw the whole weight of my body onto my left leg. I no longer stood as I had during the past year, with the toes of my right foot lightly touching the ground; instead, clutching anything within reach, or leaning against it, I let my right foot dangle aimlessly, centimetres above the floor.

Despite all my efforts to protect it, the right leg ached; sometimes the calf became numb and would sting. I cursed the damned thing, fully expecting that the next day, or definitely the day after that, the discomfort would disappear. However, it did not and I scoured the city for firm elastic supports for the ankle and knee. These did help a little, but I went on limping, stumbling and falling, while there was nothing in sight to cause me to do so.

I had been wearing the elastic guards for four days when, one morning at ten, sitting at my office desk, I became aware of a fierce pain in my right knee. It grew in intensity. I put my hand down; perhaps I had knocked the knee against a sharp edge, unwittingly cutting it, as had happened on one occasion in the past. But there was no sign of blood. I stared vaguely at my work and tried to forget that I had knees, or anything else, for that matter. But it was no good. I barely made it to the toilet before I started to rip off slacks, pantihose and the knee guard, which was now biting like a thumbscrew. I choked with relief, regarding my knee with bemusement. Strangely enough, it actually looked exactly as it always did, though now there was the delicate imprint of the elastic. I gazed and gazed at it. Not a single bruise in the vicinity. I explored around it, tentatively, with an index finger; it did not even *feel* sore. I began to dig into it more vigorously. There was no pain whatsoever. I gave up. By midday the limp was acute.

The next day – Friday, 1st August, 1975 – is branded into my memory, deeply, clearly. I did not know it then, but it marked the beginning of a time, not yet ended, which has given me poignant personal insight into some of the infinite and subtle connotations of physical pain. The limp was pronounced. Towards midday there were marked twinges low in the back. They spread, like tentacles, into the right of the rump. A strip across the lower third of both buttocks, from far left to far right, seemed chafed, and I became increasingly uncomfortable, constantly shifting my position from one side of the chair to the other. At about 2 p.m. the toes and ankle and heel of the right foot began to ache in a numb sort of way. Later, I came to call this my weeping pain: there were times when I could get no relief from it during all my waking hours; I wanted to weep, wretchedly, miserably, and once I did. The knee seared: my screaming pain, which screams could never vanquish. The lower spine flared spasmodically and sometimes, though not often, the agony swept upward, above the waist: my gasping pain, electric charges briefly but intensely felt.

These sensations, sometimes experienced alone, but more generally in concert, were to consume all my energy in the weeks to come, so that while I obediently ate whatever was put in front of me, and kept it down, my weight plunged in the first thirty days from 52 to 47 kilos, from 47 to 43. A further three kilos slipped away rather more slowly.

But on that Friday I had no inkling of what lay ahead. I stood up – and screamed. From the lower vertebrae of the spinal cord to the tip of the big toe of my right foot, I was on fire. The area from the sole of my foot, now host to a thousand sharp, penetrating pins, to just above the knee was the most badly affected by the scorch. Of the thigh only the inner surface burned. Much later, when the burn (but not the pain) became symmetrical, affecting each leg in exactly the same way, I became consciously bandy, to prevent any irritating contact between the thighs. There also seemed to be a great deal of activity in the right calf and knee, although there was only mild local pain in the latter. A thong ran up the back of the calf, binding ankle to knee. Sometimes, when this was flexible, I walked fairly easily, until it contracted and stiffened, preventing further activity – and, thank God, driving sensitivity into numbness. But on that day

56

its effect was crippling and I could barely make it over the ten me-
tres from the desk in my study to my bed.

There was little, if any, change during the week-end. On nine
separate occasions on Monday, Tuesday and Wednesday I tried to
contact Green on the phone. On five of these occasions I called at
times that had been specified by either one or the other of two women in his surgery. On the Tuesday afternoon I was obliged to excuse myself twice from the same lecture in order to do so. I thus
inconvenienced thirty adults who had paid high fees for their
course, in order to attend to personal matters. Green, however, sat
incommunicado at the other end of the line with one patient in his
room. On at least four occasions I heard the internal connection between the switchboard operator and Green being made.

The tenor of all the calls, except two, were the same. I knew the
one woman by name, but I did not identify the other, although
there would have been no difficulty in doing so since the most frequently used word in her vocabulary was "dearie". Both told me
Green was *fearfully* busy and *dreadfully* behind schedule; he could
not be disturbed. Would I call back later? If I phoned in the morning, the witching hour was 2.15; in the afternoon it was around
11.30 the next day.

At 11.30 on Tuesday 5th Miss Jones answered my call.

"Sorry, Mrs. Birrer, he's not in."

"I must speak to him. Apart from anything else, I have an
appointment for another EEG at 2.30 tomorrow. I don't know
whether to cancel it or not."

There was a prolonged pause. "Wait a minute, please."

I heard her buzz an internal connection. Seconds later she came
back to me.

"Mrs. Birrer, you need not have the EEG."

"Did Dr. Green say so?"

"Yes."

"So he is there. Please put me through – I must speak to him."

"No, I can't interrupt him."

"But you have just done so. I am quite capable of asking my
own questions, you know. Please, I have a few urgent queries, it
won't take two seconds."

"Try again at 2.15."

I did, with as little success, and yet again at 4.30. I requested Miss
Jones to ask Green to return my call the following day.

He did not. Late on Wednesday, 6th August, the other woman, who, I think, was also a bit desperate, suggested that if I *really* wanted to *speak* to Green, I make An Appointment.

"All right. Give me an appointment."

"September 26th."

"Do you know, I might be *dead* by then. I don't think so, but I might."

"Oh, *dearie,* he's going On Holiday."

So much for reporting back on the effects of Tegretol, let alone anything else.

11

I have before me as I write a standard brochure on Tegretol issued by its manufacturers. It says – note, and note well – that medical supervision during treatment is essential. It also says that blood counts should be performed regularly, that is, weekly during the first month of treatment, and monthly thereafter. This is probably because the drug *can* cause depression of bone marrow, although the incidence of this is rare. But to this very day Green does not know how the drug affected me, because he never inquired and because I was never permitted to speak to him in this connection. In the end, I relied on my family doctor to regulate the dosage, at first because the side effect of extreme drowsiness did not disappear spontaneously, and later, In November, when Green would neither accept nor return my telephone call. There seemed then to be nothing that I could do to help myself except increase the Tegretol intake to the maximum I could tolerate. I swallowed the pills as if they were jujubes. Unlike those innocuous sweets, however, the drug literally blew my mind. I felt like a zombie and I am sure that everyone who came into contact with me at the time thought I was one.

The brochure also states that Tegretol may lengthen the patient's reaction time and that this impairs safety as a road user or as an operator of machines. If, during this period, I had had an accident, causing the death of a member of the public, who should have gone on trial for culpable homicide?

When a physician writes a prescription, he is in effect silently saying to the patient: "I will take care of you." It is a promise, a pledge between the doctor and his patient. In bygone days an important aspect of this relationship was the strict obligation for the doctor to survey the drug market to ensure that no harmful or inferior ingredients were compounded in the prescription dispensed by the apothecary. With the transfer of drug production to the factory, the doctor's duty of care in this respect has increased markedly. Whether he likes it or not, he has become an unofficial salesman for an industry that is aggressively geared to financial gain.

The Thalidomide tragedy in Europe has made us acutely aware that a drug that is known to be dangerous may nevertheless be marketed, and that its detrimental effect may be recognised for some time before steps are taken to withdraw it. In general, the patient has no appreciation of incipient danger when he swallows a pill. When he does so on the authority of a prescription, any risk is transferred to the professional judgment and conscientious concern of his doctor. Thus the pill the patient swallows, no matter what its nature, acquires potency as a symbol of the faith the patient has in the doctor's wisdom, of the support he expects to receive from him. This is at the very heart of successful medical practice.

Thus the point is not merely that such an act of flagrant professional irresponsibility as that of Green constitutes a threat to life, that of the patient and those of others; even more critical is the fact that the cumulative force of these daily acts of human indifference lacerates the fabric of our existence, pillaging our lives of meaning, alienating us from ourselves and from the other.

On Thursday, 6th August, I got my hands on a large – and illegitimate – supply of Stopayne to get me through an overloaded schedule during the next fortnight. The pain did seem to subside a little, but the burning did not. My left side was holding steady; I dragged through the days, crawling into bed as soon as I could every evening. We cancelled all our engagements and I concentrated on the struggle from 8 a.m. to 8 p.m., and on staying sane.

On Wednesday, 27th August, the pain began in earnest. If the Stopayne was working at all, it was not doing a very good job. Six weeks had passed since the angiogram. I tried a bit of elementary logic.

I do not have a brain tumour.

I do have a Chiari.

59

Therefore my pain is due to the Chiari.

The pain, of course, was something quite apart from the burning, but then I had not been given the opportunity to report this development. But the burn aside, if this kind of pain was what having a Chiari meant, I was no longer so sure that I could manage. In fact, I needed help, other than the surgical variety. I needed tougher pain killers to tide me over, although I was not enthusiastic about that idea either. But a Chiari fluctuates. All I had to do was buy a bit of time; this sticky patch would pass.

I thought the best way to handle the matter was to see my G.P. Probably I should have done so long before. I doubted that Green would refuse to speak to a colleague nine times in a row.

But as the weeks passed I began to suspect – call it a woman's intuition – that this had been a large assumption to make. I know that my general practitioner did speak to Green, several times, but I doubt that he found it easy to do so, although he never said as much. I have heard that the task is beyond many doctors.

This is hearsay, of course, but one story at least so closely resembles my own that to my mind it bears the stamp of authenticity. It is from a patient who has the same disease as I have, and who had the same neurologist. A few months ago, the patient's ophthalmologist found that the pressure in the eyes was excessive, and the specialist physician found on lumbar puncture that the pressure of the spinal fluid was over 300 (a pressure of 150 mm water is considered normal[1]). The patient made more attempts "than there are fingers on both hands" to contact Green. These efforts did eventually meet with success, although the patient was accused of "persecution". Nonetheless, Green saw his tormentor, denied that there was any undue intra-ocular pressure and insisted that if the patient had any problems at all, they were due to marital difficulties.

Be that as it may, the patient felt unable to cope with Green and asked the general practitioner to try and get some sense out of him. He, too, failed hopelessly, because Green simply refused to answer the telephone. Since patient and G. P. both live elsewhere on the Reef, there was no question of storming the bastion. This doctor now refers to Green as "that little tin god".

My general practitioner had seen me on and off over several

1. Conybeare, J. (Ed.): *Textbook of Medicine.* Edinburgh, E. & S. Livingstone Ltd., 1947.

years, but apart from fairly regular bouts of 'flu and bronchitis, as well as annual attacks of hay fever during the first quarter of each year, I had been symptom-free ever since 1960, when Professor Jansen of the University of Cape Town performed an operation to rectify a pyloric stenosis. This is a constriction of the end of the stomach that opens into the first part of the duodenum, and it prevents the passage of food and (eventually, in my case) liquids.

I saw Dr. Rice for the first time in connection with my current problems on 13th August. Apart from my neurological difficulties, he said, there was some local inflammation in the knee. I left with a prescription for Tanderil to counteract this development, and his promise to discuss matters with Green. He did so. There was nothing Green could find, apart from the Chiari, to account for the things I was complaining about. I saw or phoned Rice on alternate days until the school holidays intervened. The Tanderil made no noticeable difference to the pain in the knee, and there was definitely no change in the condition of my back and the rest of my legs.

On 3rd September Dr. Peters, a radiologist, X-rayed the lower lumbar region and reported a hint of prolapsis in two discs. On 5th September I passed the information on to Green - miraculously, over the phone. He seemed relieved that a surgical sickness might be present to explain away the pain and burn I was now ranting about. He would see me if I insisted (but he didn't know when), or maybe Mr. Aschen could see me; that was a *much better* idea. But the most sensible one of all was fourteen days' bed-rest.

During this conversation I felt that now I really was sinking into a vortex. What had happened to the double vision? What did the fits mean? Was I going permanently lame? Why had I suddenly developed a pain in the lower part of my back? I did not believe for a fleeting second that one vertebra had prolapsed, let alone two. I was able to move around the waist in ways no slipped disc would have allowed. My biggest problem was the fact that Green seemed to have lost sight of the over-all picture; or, if he had not, it was all due to that incorrigible Chiari throwing up symptoms.

Well, nearly all, anyway. This conversation also sowed the seed of a suspicion that Green was not only keeping the neurological back door wide open, but was also looking for other exits.

"I am having very painful attacks of pins and needles in both hands and both feet."

"You must be hyperventilating."

"I am not hyperventilating."

"You must be."

Four courses were open to me: insist on seeing Green, and he had actively discouraged this; insist on seeing Aschen; go to bed for fourteen days; carry on - which I did, or tried to do. But there are limits to what the mind can demand of the body. On Tuesday, 9th September, I collapsed, lame. My right leg could not bear my weight, nor move to my command. I was mad with pain and burn; now I could not tell, nor did I care, which was which.

12

One week melted into the next. The pain tore into the flesh, stripping a little from the bones each day; it dulled the wits, so that the daily newspapers became a serious intellectual challenge; it weakened the will, though it never quite crushed it. I wanted to be up, away from that austere room with its white stucco plaster and wooden rockers. But the pain resisted everything: it remained untouched by Valoron, Doloxene, DF118. There was no elixir, no relief until, fortuitously, I received a small but adequate supply of Pethidine pills. I took three and knew I had to get rid of them, that the cure could prove worse than the disease - whatever it was. In a moment of uncharacteristic strength I flushed them down the loo. I was watching my life blood swill away in the turbulence, so desperate was my need for the respite they offered. I finally settled for 600 mg of Doloxene per day; although it made no impressive impact on the degree of pain I was experiencing, at least I did not become nauseous on it.

I grew drawn and pale, hair stringy and unusually greasy from the eternal twisting and turning against green striped pillows that became damp and hot and creased. I supposed ruefully that this was how Jill thought I should look when I saw Green. "Whenever you see him you look as though you've had a holiday," she said furiously, staring at my freshly washed hair as I slipped into the front seat of her car one day. Bill had also once, before a dinner date, glanced at me, sparkling outwardly and shrunken inwardly, and remarked that it was difficult to believe that I was ill. But I do not see a doctor unless I have a tale to tell. Do I have to look like a hag in order to be believed?

The pain scourged my body, sapped my mind. That was bad enough. But with equal ferocity it flayed those who cared. Bill also had to live through those excruciating night hours when I could not lie on my back, or stand, or walk, or bend, when I could barely move my limbs at all, when I could not tolerate the merest pressure of a sheet, or of night wear, or of bed socks, against the skin of back and limb and upper instep; when all he saw was me shrouded in misery, and he could do nothing, nothing but bring another glass of water and another Doloxene. He became irascible, tenser, thinner. My parents too saw most of it, keeping steadfastly cheerful as they fetched and carried, but inwardly fuming, fretting, breaking their hearts a little more each day. My friends saw a great deal of it, keeping in constant contact by telephone, arriving gay and leaving grey.

On 26th September I kept the appointment with Green that I had with so much difficulty made more than a month and a half previously. Drugged, in great pain, weak from bed-rest and rapid loss of weight, I remember very little. He dug his thumb into the flesh beneath my big right toe. I yelped.

"*Ah-ha!* What *you* need is a good orthopod. This pain can be fixed easily, with a metatarsal bar in your shoe. We'll get onto that."

The leg was in spasm. Green thought that was due to whatever Myodil remained in the spine from the myelogram he had done on 28th January. Arrangements were made to remove the Myodil the following day. About the addition to my foot-gear I said nothing. I knew from experience I would not be seeing an orthopaedic surgeon, not on Green's initiative anyway.

Green said that as far as he was concerned there was no sign of prolapsis in the lumbar region on the X-rays Peters had taken. The next day, 27th September, the myelogram was rescreened to confirm this.

"There is nothing there. I told you so," said he, sanctimoniously, setting my teeth on edge. I was trapped face downwards on the X-ray table, with Pethidine dripping slowly, blessedly, into a vein on the back of my left hand. Apart from the fact that this particular situation enforced inactivity, I scarcely had the strength to swat a fly. But my inclination was to hit him. Hard. And it had nothing to do with being crazy, either.

Green had been quite prepared to confine me to bed for the customary fourteen days for a pain that *may* have resulted from a prolapsed disc. On the other hand, it may not have had anything to do with a disc; after all, no one had ever claimed that there was more than a hint of prolapsis. He had checked neither plates nor patient to assess for himself what the cause of the pain might be. And yet, as the neurologist in charge of the case, no one knew better than he that for the preceding eighteen months I had been victim to one strange symptom after another. Even if he did think I was a raving nut (which I was beginning to suspect he did), he had not actually said so. Had he done so, I would of course have sought help elsewhere. As far as I was concerned, therefore, he was obligated to search unremittingly for some medical basis for my pathology where this appeared to exceed the limits of the early diagnosis he had fixed his mind on, as it was surely beginning to do. I did not see then, and I do not see now, how he could possibly have formed an accurate assessment of, let alone pass judgment on, my psychological state. He knew next to nothing about me as a person and he apparently understood even less about the infinite complexities of psychological growth, its resilience, its fathomless potential. To allow his psychological prevarications to bedevil his medical commitment was impudent at best, heinous at worst. If the Myodil was causing the burn, or if it was responsible for the pain in the leg, I might have been spared weeks of agony.

The Myodil came out on Saturday, 27th September, and the pain eased for twenty-four hours. I left a message of appreciation at Green's home: at least he had ensured that what is often an unpleasant procedure had been painless. I also said that I thought it had made a difference. By 6 p.m. on Sunday I knew I was mistaken. Rice phoned Green, who was surprised. Surprised. Full stop.

October was purgatory. Dr. Rice, who saw me on alternate days throughout this period, phoned Green on two or three occasions to report the lack of improvement. Friends and family pressed me daily to call for further medical opinions, but I was reluctant. I had been told that, from a neurological point of view, in Green I had The Best. Was there any sense, then, in shopping around?

Jill fumed and accused me of unfairness to everyone, including myself. Finally she resorted to sweet reasonableness. "Well, maybe you *have* got the best, but does it make any difference when you can't get him on the phone and when he seems to have lost interest in the case? If you get someone else, maybe not so good, at least you'll have something. Face it, now you've got nothing, and it's going from bad to worse."

Ann was a little more succinct: "Don't you think Green has outlived his usefulness?"

They were right. As far as neurological care was concerned, I really did seem to have nothing. And it was also true that nothing seemed to help for the pain. In desperation I tried Ronicol-Timespan, which is used for peripheral vascular disorders, and Fenopron, normally used for rheumatoid arthritis. But nothing helped: Tanderil, Ronicol, Fenopron, tranquillisers, painkillers, bed-rest at home, bed-rest in Mauritius - *nothing*. Even the good effects of Epanutin and Tegretol seemed to be evaporating, as I had on one occasion lost consciousness again.

But whatever else I do or do not suffer from, it seems I definitely have an unnatural respect for the power of the intellect. I believe passionately that intelligence shall deliver us from evil, although it is crystal clear from the state of the world we live in that I am hopelessly misled. I could not accept then that Green might be a microcosm of the macrocosm; nor was the close interdependence between medical thought and conduct and the human values prevalent in this society, as well as in the world at large, as clear to me then as it is now.

Be that as it may, I finally succumbed to the pressure. Making a last-ditch stand for my delusion, I insisted on having someone who was at least connected with the medical school at the university. I was assured that Professor Barron was the right man, and the arrangements to see him were made by a friend, who said he would put it straight with Green, who would not mind anyway, as he had a lot of respect for Barron. If not exactly birds of a feather, they were at least piping the same tune.

My husband, now a deeply worried man, phoned Green to discuss the events of the case with him. For the third time Green refused to speak to him. I had had more than I could stomach of that kind of behaviour and poured my fury into a letter. Green's reply of 6th November incensed me further. He claimed he had no idea that I still had pain, because he had not heard from me. No, he had not, for a very good reason; but since 27th September he had certainly heard from my G.P. on the subject, and more than once.

I phoned Green and was put through. He absolved himself from all responsiblity for calls that disappeared, eerily, at his switchboard, and made an appointment to see me on 15th November. I still believed he could put his finger on the problem without overtaxing himself, if only he set his mind to it.

13

I saw Professor Barron on 14th November. For the first time, Bill was with me. It was the strangest consultation I have had with any doctor; in fact, it was bizarre. I had heard Barron was eccentric; egocentric was a more apt description, I decided. We sat down facing him, a table, bare save for one small pad and a pen, between us. Perhaps there was an ashtray as well.

"Tell me what the problem is."

Well, the problem was a painful and fiery leg which often caused me to limp badly, and I tried to get this across to the figure in front of me. He leaned far back in his chair, pressing his neck back into the fingers of both hands, which were entwined, cradle-like. The winged elbows wagged gently to and fro. But he was not interested in legs, at least not mine; he wanted, or so he said, to hear the whole story *right* from the beginning. I took a deep breath and plunged into that marathon, racing a little over the events of 1974, assiduously ignoring the faint air of boredom that wafted across the desk. I stared determinedly at the wooden surface in front of me, stopping to get my second wind only when I reached the first series of fits. My listener disentangled his fingers, slouched gently sideways and reached toward the pad. It was a fraction too far. He heaved forward and tried again; his fingers slipped off the pad. It is astonishing how much effort is needed to pull a note pad across the surface of a desk, but he persisted. At last it moved toward him. He rested the lower part of his forearm and wrist on the desk and wrote two words, one under the other. Each ended with a pronounced flourish. The hand shot up and snapped backwards at the wrist, leaving the pen pointing firmly at the ceiling in a gesture of total conviction. It had the effect on me of a cobra poised to strike: hypnotic. By the end of the interview I was, in fact, in a trance.

I plodded on to the EEGs.

"Did they show anything?"

"Yes. They . . ."

"You don't have to say any more. I know the answer."

My jaw sagged. Bill later said his did too. I gurgled in astonishment, otherwise speechless.

"All right. Go on, if you want to." He beamed at Bill. "So-and-so (unknown to both of us) always said, *let* the patient talk. That way you get the *full* story."

Ten minutes had passed since the consultation began. I looked at him, my head tilted slightly to the right to make quite sure I missed nothing. Green was a pretty snappy diagnostician, but he was no match for this – unless, of course, Barron had been primed so well that nothing further really needed to be said. "He is fully conversant with the facts of your case," Green had written in his letter of 6th November. With exaggerated deliberation I scanned the desk top, left to right, right to left. I let my eyes search the few surface areas in the room. Barron watched me. He knew perfectly well what I was looking for.

"I never read a file before I see a patient," he breezed. Obviously, anyone who did was a Bloody Fool. He jabbed the air with his pen. My eyes followed it as it rose once more toward the ceiling. I stared at it sightlessly, certain in my own mind that the file had never left Green's office, or that if it had, it had been waved aside by the extraordinary creature in front of me.

In broad terms, doctors base their diagnoses on two kinds of information: hard facts, or demonstrative evidence, such as a myelogram may reveal, and soft facts. Evidence derived from sources such as myelograms exists for anyone to examine, and every doctor has access to the identical information. Soft facts are less tangible: for example, the patient's report of events such as faints or fits. These are often personal, in that they have not been witnessed by anyone else. However, in both cases information becomes *fact* when it is understood and interpreted. This can only occur within the conceptual framework that the individual doing the interpreting has developed through training and experience. A temperature of 39°C, as measured by the mercury of a thermometer, may be a hard "fact", but it is meaningless without a conception of how mercury expands with heat, and of how a rise in temperature relates to the physical state of the body.

Obviously no two doctors can ever have the same frame of reference. Thus, given identical information, two neurologists may reach quite diverse opinions. I know of no case that illustrates this more starkly than my own. This flexibility is a two-edged sword: on the one hand, it may introduce conflict between doctors, and undue stress for the patient; on the other, old facts seen in a new and quite different perspective may considerably advance understanding of the patient's problem. To be of value, therefore, the reinterpretation demands impartiality in the specialist who has been approached to make it.

However, it seemed that here the "facts" in Barron's possession had already been thoroughly conceptualised by Green. But even if Barron did have the file, I was equally sure that it would be returned unopened. Nothing Barron reported back to Green would be tainted by his first-hand acquaintance with hard neurological evidence, nor would the soft stuff be really rethought and freshly digested. I sniffed a strong aroma of trouble.

The pen clattered noisily onto the desk. I jumped. Barron flicked the note pad around with the élan of a croupier.

"I knew it, of course. Look here, I've noted it down."

We both leaned forward. The list had grown to five or six words, and one of them was "temporal". He underlined it with his index finger. "That's your problem. Temporal lobe." What he meant, but did not say, was "epilepsy of the temporal lobe".

I looked at the man. I hung my head. No wonder there is so much public support for the anti-applause-for-academics league. I wanted to pay for whatever service Barron felt he had rendered and walk out. But I was seeing him at my urgent request, and though I now realised my choice was a tactical error that could have unfortunate repercussions, I supposed I had to see it through.

Bill and I both made several efforts to steer the conversation away from the subject of epilepsy, which Barron insisted on pursuing. I tried repeatedly to slip in a report of the development of events subsequent to the series of attacks in which he was so interested, but which had not recurred since I had begun taking Tegretol. But he would have none of it. He launched into a splendid, if patronising, dissertation on the social consequences of epilepsy, taking great pains to assure me that no mental disorder any longer carries the stigma it once did. For fifteen minutes I listened to a straight rerun of many of the points I take pains to make to students who are beginning their teaching careers and who may for the first time come into contact with an epileptic child. My fears and anxieties, he said, were quite unfounded; my friends were my friends, and I'd soon find out who they were.

Now I wanted to open my mouth and scream. My friends are indeed my friends, and I doubt whether there is *any* woman who is more aware of the fact, or of how lucky she is. On my first stay in Lords Nursing Home I had been in a two-bed ward with a pleasant companion who had been in and out of hospitals for more than eighteen months. She had confided that the previous month she had taken her nine-year-old son out of school.

"You mean, for good?"

"No; for the time being."

"You can't do that; for one thing, it's illegal."

"Well, I'm not allowed to drive and there's no bus service where we are. But we are trying to sell the house, and move nearer the school, but its difficult . . ."

"Your friends - won't they . . .?"

"Well, I dunno. I think they're fed up with me being sick all the time."

I had risked a post-lumbar-puncture hangover and turned to look at her. Human flotsam, awash in the high tide of cruel circumstance.

During the wretched period that began in January 1974 my friends have fetched me, chauffeured me in and outside of Johannesburg, shopped for me, tracked down the *last* artichoke, or the *first* cherry of the season, cooked for me - the pâtés and pizzas and pastries I love - and scoured library shelves for me. And they do this, and much more, not once a month, or once a week, but every single day, and there have been more than seven hundred and thirty such days. I *know,* without being assured or reassured by anyone at all, that they will continue to do so for as long as they feel I need their help.

I have a family and I *know* about them, too. I have an exceptional husband who, no doubt foolishly, believes I am a pearl beyond price. There is nothing within reason - and that covers a wide range by anybody's standards - that he would not get for me or do for me. My parents would lay down their lives for mine, and express their devotion in countless deeds every day of my life.

I also had a job, and I *knew* about that, too. During 1975 the Head of the Department of Education showed me nothing but consideration and kindness, even at those times when my disability caused serious inconvenience to himself and to the staff and students. Outside the confines of my family and a close circle of friends, very little has been said about my health problems. I have never discussed them with any member of the university staff. When my absences from the campus became more frequent, I knew that dozens of rumours were flying around. I heard some wild ones, but commented on none. One day, when I walked into a lecture room through a back door, every head swung round, eyes riveted to my waistline. Afterwards a student who was also a friend begged me to assure the others that I was not pregnant, since it was widely known that I was living alone. There did not seem much point in that, since all they had to do was wait a few months and their worst - or best - fears would be confirmed. I also did not want to spoil the delicious sense of anticipation some of them must have felt.

Colleagues with whom I worked closely obviously knew I was ill. I did what I could to maintain the quality of my lecturing, although the quantity rapidly tailed off to nothing. But I could not function intellectually while I was in so much pain. Besides that, my concentration had been flagging for some time, although I forced myself to do some writing and to complete a degree, using increasingly refined mnemonic devices to assuage the apparent onslaught of Tegretol on my memory.

Throughout all this I felt the support of the departmental head, and as I limped through the year I derived great comfort from the knowledge that the opportunity existed to return to participate in the rituals of academic life.

And, of course, I have a past. Looking back over it I find nothing to regret. An aunt once said (rather grudgingly, I have always thought) that I had been born with a gold spoon in my mouth. And really, I have lived a charmed life. There have been crises, of course, but these have not been destructive: they constitute important growth points in my life, which have led into new and different channels. Through the years this has given my life an enduring quality of freshness. I have done the best I could at each turning point, and - at least as far as I am concerned - the results have always been worthwhile.

One major crisis was largely due, as the present one is, to a retreat by members of the medical profession in the face of a physical ailment they could not comprehend; a retreat to a bottomless chasm which reverberates with the echoes of the shattering conclusions of

70

Sigmund Freud, now reduced to an ideology, a bundle of barbs with a lethal sting. But that cloud proved to have a lining of sterling quality, and so, I believe, will this one.

Looking at Barron then, I marvelled. We heard him out because there was nothing else we could do. I reminded him, without any hope that he would make some positive contribution towards a solution, that my leg constituted a problem to the degree that it was seriously interfering with ordinary day-to-day living. He indicated that I should go behind the screened area in the corner of the room. I did so and removed my slacks. He followed me.

"Oh no, there was no need for that. Never mind."

He did not touch my spine and he barely looked at my legs. In all we were behind the curtain for approximately three minutes.

When I came back to the desk he was looking at the X-rays. I asked whether he thought I had a Chiari.

"No, you haven't got a Chiari. I don't believe in Chiaris. I'm too old-fashioned. I leave that to the boys at Lords Nursing Home."

I had told the friend-who-made-the-arrangements that I wanted a realistic assessment of the Chiari. Now I mentally divided Johannesburg into two with an invisible line running north to south. The boys in the west believe in a congenital anomaly of the hindbrain; the boys in the east do not. In other words, in order to have a Chiari you have to choose the right geographical location. But maybe Barron had meant something else: the boys in the west are congenital idiots; the boys in the east are not. You just pay your money and take your chance.

He picked up the most recent X-rays, those of the lower lumbar region.

"But of course Peters is right."

"You think there is prolapsis?"

"Yes."

"*Two* discs?"

"Yes. Does warmth help?"

"It has been known to."

"Of course it does. Is it painful to ride in a car?"

"Sometimes, very."

He was clearly anxious to leave. He assured us, heartily, that the leg was Quite All Right, nothing at all to worry about. He would Let Green Know What the Matter Was.

71

We thanked him. I lowered my head, lifting my eyelids just enough for one last, long look. I thought he was, among other things, the most bombastic man I had ever met. At that particular moment I did not care whether he told Green I was as mad as a March hare, or whether he did not. It was getting more and more like the Mad Hatter's tea party, anyway.

14

Seated in the car again, with one arm slung across the steering wheel, the other draped along the back of the front seat, Bill turned to me, puzzled.

What, he inquired, was all that about?

He had not detected the catastrophic course upon which I had been set, but I certainly had. I had been caught completely off guard and left nonplussed. I had been unable to gather my wits quickly enough to counter the conclusions which were clearly assembled in Barron's mind. He had decided with lightning speed that the problem I was experiencing with my leg was a hysterical reaction to an ungrounded anxiety about epilepsy which had, just as quickly, achieved quite extraordinary dimensions. I was struck dumb. But in any event protest would have been bootless. When a decision is reached that behaviour is a hysterical reaction, there is practically nothing to be said or done. Contrary claims vehemently expressed only serve to entrench ill-founded conviction.

I was astonished by my own naïvete. But I *was* also worried. Barron's unfortunate opinion was of consequence only in so far as Green was influenced by it, but I could not judge to what extent he would be. I strongly suspected that it would tip the balance of the scales in favour of a tawdry psychological cliché, since he seemed to be in danger of running out of neurological signs. I was sick, and I had been sick for a very long time. Now I was thoroughly weakened by pain. Although I was a bit low on occasion, and had once been given tranquillisers by Rice, there had been no depression. Nevertheless my resistance was paper thin; the stiff upper lip had begun to quiver. There seemed to be little doubt that my problems were neurological, and – terrifying thought – I was dependent on

72

Green to resolve them. What other course lay open? I knew I could seek help elsewhere, in South Africa or overseas, but I was tired. Suddenly, tired unto death. What was it all about, anyway?

With a sense of deep foreboding I kept my appointment with Green, arriving promptly at 11 a.m. on Saturday, 15th November. Green arrived at approximately 11.10 a.m. He had, he said, just seen Barron. I started. My file was in front of him, and yet when he arrived I had thought he was empty-handed. So Barron *had* made a diagnosis on a diagnosis.

What did I think, Green asked? I thought Barron had missed the point altogether, and I said so as forcefully as I could. He was convinced I was deeply concerned about the social implications of my unfortunate affliction – fear and anxiety, he said, those are the invariable characteristics of an epileptic. Naturally I had felt fear during the period of the head explosions. But my fear had been wholly concerned with the damage they might be doing to my brain. I have never suffered any anxiety about fits, certainly not in the sense of being embarrassed about their occurring in a restaurant or cinema. Frankly, it had never crossed my mind that I should feel that way. Whatever for? I cannot help my fits, and every precaution that I know of has been taken to bring them under control. Until very recently this has apparently been successful. If I passed out in a restaurant and a fellow diner was upset, *he* had a problem, not I. If I did so at a social gathering – well, I did, as Barron said, know my friends. Today there is little enough time left in every twenty-four hours for fun and amusement; Bill and I agree in that we are not prepared to spend that precious residue with people we do not care about. No, during the months when the faints or fits were prevalent we did not once cancel a social engagement; we entertained and were entertained as before. But my leg was a horse of quite a different colour; apart from ten days in Mauritius, where I spent more time in bed than on the beach, and a disastrous foray to a new restaurant in Bryanston, I never left the house for more than an hour at any one time.

That particular night is one four of us will never forget. It began with a glass of wine and snacks at 7.30 p.m. in the home of our hosts. We went on in high spirits to enjoy the décor and old-world cuisine of a new restaurant. At about 10 p.m., when friends came over to the table for a word with the men, I took the opportunity to slip out to the cloak-room. I remember leaving the table, but nothing more.

My absence was only noticed when the threesome turned back to their rare beef and yorkshire pudding. Deanna found me spread-eagled on the floor near the hand-basins. It was the first time I had passed out since beginning the Tegretol.

My first recollection is of lying on the back seat of the car, my head on Deanna's lap. The engine started and the car moved forward. It is one of the starkest memories of my life. A massive electric charge swept the entire length of my spine, from base to neck. I screamed and turned my head to one side. Tearing, searing pain coursed through the neck, scorching every membrane of my scalp, although there was no pain *in* the head itself. I screamed again, swinging my head involuntarily to the other side. Head and neck were excoriated: I was a human dynamo, discharging volt after volt along the spine and over the surface of the head. It seemed to me that there had to be an ultimate explosion, that the vertebrae must rip through the skin and be spewed far and wide into the night. Charge followed charge, moan followed moan. The car stopped and started and stopped again. Every loose piece of clothing was wedged around my hips and waist. Deanna gripped my head between her large, strong hands; Gary leaned over the front seat, trying to help me retain a rigid position. It took Bill two hours to cover the few kilometres home.

In the bedroom I swallowed the last handful of Doloxene and Gary went out to scour the neighbourhood pharmacies for more. Bill filled the bath with hot water and Deanna supported my floating body until about 3 a.m., when the pain receded and I began to feel sleepy. Tucked in at last, I fell into a slumber from which I fervently prayed I would never wake.

Now I also told Green that Barron had said Peters was right about the prolapsed discs. I was watching him closely. His murmured "yes" did not give much away, and he motioned me to the side room. I went in and undressed. He examined the leg from foot to lower spine, very thoroughly.

I was lying on my left side, staring at the wall. He seemed to be a little perplexed, but not unduly so.

"The hip *is* in spasm. And if it's in spasm, it must be reacting to something."

"Of course it's reacting to something. You don't have this kind of

74

pain unless there is something to react to."

I glanced over my shoulder as I spoke. I had seen him like that only once before, when my right arm had taken on a life of its own: moving instruments on his table, face darkened, slightly slouched forward, concentrating.

"That is not so. You can have great pain when nothing is organically wrong." He spoke very quietly.

I froze, still looking at him over my shoulder. My heart sank. It was the first clear indication that the great retreat was under way, the withdrawal of the embattled physician under pretext of neurasthenia, hypochondriasis, neuroses, hysteria - you name it, the doctor has got it in his armamentarium of defences against unidentifiable organic and metabolic pathologies, the bricks and mortar of the medical practitioner's own personal fortification, his impregnable Sigfreud Line.

No, I thought, no, no, no. He *is* too good a neurologist to fall into that trap. *Where* did this case come unstuck? And then I looked back at the wall and thought about the Moravian Jew who in the early years of this century had transformed man's conception of himself. I marvelled, as I have so many times in my life, at the invincible power an idea can have. The most pervasive force in human life is, and ever will be, an idea, and the generative concepts that have fructified each age of man are indestructible. But sometimes they calcify and become retrograde in their effect. And since we are so rarely aware of the invisible forces that suffuse the spirit we, too, calcify and become mere marionettes. We are no longer regenerated and enriched by the idea, but become subservient to and impoverished by the ideology.

Green stood behind me with the X-rays of the lower spine in his left hand, ball-point in his right, and a truculent expression on his face. Holding the negatives above his head, he let his pen follow the outline of the lower lumbar discs.

"Look, if any of these were prolapsed it would look like this . . ." He traced an imaginary bulge below that on the X-ray. I could have been looking at Scotch mist, but in this case I was sure he was right. "*But* I'm not saying you haven't got disc problems - off the X-ray. And maybe one of the discs is vrot. I think you ought to have a discogram. Ll - a disc in the lumbar region of the spine."

Well, I knew that this was one procedure radiologists are not enthusiastic about, as it entails injecting a dye into the disc prior to

X-raying it. Nor was I willing to have another needle jabbed into my spine, particularly when there was some doubt as to whether it was necessary. I said so and he went out.

I slipped off the bed and into my clothes. My mind was racing. I was fighting for my health and losing ground all the time. What could I do to salvage the situation? I went and sat in the chair opposite Green.

"I want another opinion."

His eyes, merry, widened.

"Who did you have in mind?"

I had not expected to have to take this step and had to think for a moment. I mentioned a name.

"He'll chuck you out. He'll think you're mad."

We stared at each other. What went through his mind I do not know; I gasped. He noticed it.

"You would be better off with either Brown or Kenny."

I knew of Kenny, that he was highly regarded, and that he had wide experience.

"Give me the one with a few grey hairs."

He laughed and lifted the phone.

"Please make an appointment with Mr. Kenny for a third, fourth, fifth opinion for Mrs. Birrer." He chuckled.

I looked at him grimly. I was glad he was in such good spirits. As far as I was concerned there was nothing at all, not one single thing, to be amused about. If necessary there would be a sixth, seventh, eighth opinion. Life is for living, and nothing on this earth is going to stop me from doing so, if I can help it.

I left the room. Outside I stopped. Maybe, I thought wearily, maybe there is just a grain of truth in what he thinks. I went back.

"Please give me a script for Serepax 15."

For four days I took the tranquillisers at four-hourly intervals. On the fifth they went the way of the Pethidine, only not for the same reason. There was no point in swallowing drugs that had no effect.

15

The following Tuesday, 18th November, I hobbled into Mr. Kenny's surgery. He exchanged a few pleasantries with Bill and we all sat down. At least they did. I eased myself delicately into a firmly upholstered maroon chair, relieved when the task was successfully accomplished. For no reason at all I glanced over my shoulder; my eyes fell on a long, low cupboard against the wall. I had the identical one in my dining room at home. Well, at least he had good taste. But I gave him a stony stare. I was as wary as a cat on a midnight prowl; would this experience be as futile and disastrous as the last? It was difficult to tell. He was not young, but neither was he old. And he kept his eyes down, not actually avoiding my gaze, but with an air of professional reticence that seemed as natural to him as breathing. Was he his own man? Could he make up his own mind, form an opinion for himself? That was all I asked of him.

This time I did not try to gallop through any period in the development of my problems. I had thought it all through carefully, trying to husband the facts as faithfully as possible. But he ferreted out a good deal more, questioning closely, deftly. Now he often glanced at me intently through his spectacles. Once or twice we stared hard at each other, each weighing up the other.

At the end of the interview he remarked that, of course, Green knew me better than he did. I felt inclined to disagree. It seemed to me that both *knew* me as well as any specialist can ever really get to know a patient in the course of a professional consultation, or even a series of these. Green was certainly aware, in addition, that I had been left unperturbed by a myelogram and angiogram, and even during the conduct of the latter – or, at least, I was then. Today payment in gold would not persuade me to submit to either procedure under any but the most extraordinary circumstances. He also knew that I did not raise hell when confined to bed in a nursing home, although many situations I encountered while I was there called for raising hell: the quality of patient care in Lords Nursing Home is a public scandal. And, to heap insult on injury, "You *have* to go there; nowhere else." But these disconnected snippets of information do not constitute the royal road to an insightful grasp of the human personality, even in the hands of a man psychologically more astute than Green. In fact, Green had travelled down a few blind alleys and now he seemed to be within skidding distance of a complete cul de sac.

Kenny found out where I was born and something of my early life and medical problems. Together we traced the sequence of events during 1974 and 1975, while he painstakingly recorded the history of my misery from the first attack of double vision to the racking pains of the previous evening. He asked me whether there had been deterioration in my speech and whether my concentration had wavered at any time. He wanted to know what neurological procedures had been undertaken; had I had an EMI scan? No. I had not. The equipment for this had only recently been installed at a local nursing home. In essence, an EMI is a brain scan in which X-raying is combined with a computer print-out. The information this provides obviates the necessity for, among other things, an angiogram and an air encephalogram (where an EEG reading is taken after the introduction of air into the head). The procedure involves lying motionless for anything up to an hour with the top of the head encased in a hairdryer-like contraption with a rubbery, water-filled lining to ensure a snug fit. The scan costs approximately R180, but it does eliminate the risks which inhere in the procedures it replaces.

Kenny made it clear that he did not think the scan would reveal anything new. "But can you afford to leave any stone unturned when your difficulties are proliferating daily?"

Kenny went back to probing those difficulties. Did I urinate frequently; was there any urgency to do so? Was I always as unsteady on my feet? What? Where? When . . .?

I watched him study the X-rays.

"You know, don't you, that you do have a cerebellar tonsil?"

"Yes, Mr. Aschen was called in to see me just after the myelogram was done."

"Did he suggest any operation?"

"No. He more or less rejected the idea out of hand. It seemed too equivocal."

"Of course. I do not think it can possibly account for your problems."

He examined me. The same tests: eyes, pin-pricks from the crown of my head to the tips of my toes, touching my nose and his finger alternately, recognition of objects placed in my hand, reflexes, and so on. As far as I could judge the results in all respects were the same as those Green had obtained in his first examination in January, with the exception that there was now no instance of double vision. I found it very difficult to resist the pressure on my right knee from Kenny's hand, but I did not think that he thought there was any significant difference between the legs, or any weakness in either.

Thoroughly alerted to the possibility of a prolapsed disc, he checked and rechecked for the relevant signs.

"I can find no indication of a disc problem."

I dressed and joined the silent couple in the adjoining room. Kenny looked up from his pad and remarked on the complexity of the case. He promised that he and Green would put their heads together and work something out.

It was a job well done; the conduct of the entire examination was immaculate. I thought that if he did not make something of it, probably nobody could.

We all stood up. I looked at Kenny. "Do you think it is anything sinister?"

He paused, impassive, and looked me straight in the eye.

"Mrs. Birrer, you have got problems." He placed no emphasis on any of his words.

As we got to the door, I asked whether cortisone might not help to settle the burn. "I think ACTH would be better in your case," was his response. ACTH, or adrenocorticotropic hormone, stimulates the production of cortisone by the body.

On the way home I thought it all over. Three things had emerged: Kenny did think I was ill; he did not think that the Chiari had much, if anything, to do with it; and he certainly did not think that I had prolapsed discs. I had got the impression that he thought a degenerative factor was operative in the nervous system, though I did not know what name he would give it. What I did know, without any shadow of doubt, was that it was a diagnosis Green would not accept. He had his own views on the matter and he seemed less and less willing to change or modify them as time went by. I fully expected to hear from him that he had a difference of opinion with Kenny, and that he would therefore recommend another medical opinion.

Bill shot a red light and turned to me. "I have no idea when a case is complex and when it is not, but I reckon you have to be a genius to sort that lot out."

On Friday morning my husband called Green to find out what had transpired. Green's receptionist informed him Bill was on the phone, but Green refused to speak to him. The conversation between Green and his employee was audible at the other end of the line. The message that Bill finally received was a request for me to phone the surgery at 2.15 that afternoon.

I did so. "Have you discussed the case with Mr. Kenny?"

"Yes." The voice was short and had an indifferent ring I had not heard before, and somewhere I detected a touch of defiance.

"What did he say?"

"Kenny can find nothing wrong with you." Obviously there were no geniuses around. The silence began to ring in my ears. "He is not prepared to touch either your neck or your spine. He wants you to have an EMI scan, but I think it's gilding the lily. Do you want it? It costs money . . ."

"Yes, of course I'll have it."

"O.K. Yes, I suppose you may as well."

"Look, I am in pain, very great pain, and I am on fire. Will you give me cortisone to settle the burn?"

"I can find no neurological sign for the cortisone to work on. It would be a pharmacological assault on the system. I won't do it."

"What about the pain?"

"Well, I still think a discogram . . ."

"Kenny, you yourself and the radiologist who rescreened the myelogram all think that there is no disc problem. Why do I need a discogram?"

"Well, I don't know . . . I could increase the Tegretol, I suppose . . ."

"What about the Chiari?"

"I still think it's there."

I put the phone down. For the first time I wondered seriously whether there was not a thread of psychological imbalance woven into the case. The man at the other end of the line was obsessive. I mean, anyone would think he had invented the Chiari. Or maybe he suffered from a severe and unnatural fear of being wrong, or from an unnatural unconcern for patients with peculiar pathologies. Actually, there were a lot of things he could be suffering from – after all, what is sauce for the goose is certainly sauce for the gander.

But my thoughts quickly turned away from the mental staleness and ennui of the rigidified mind infatuated with a single idea to the immediate problem. What on earth was I going to do with a crippled leg and a body that burned continually, occasionally flaring into an inferno? Eventually I decided to keep my cool and push up the dose of Tegretol myself. On that day I slipped in two extra pills: one with my afternoon tea and one later, on going to sleep. The following day, Saturday, I doubled the dose: two each before breakfast, lunch and dinner. I took another at bed time. On Sunday I repeated the same dosage.

Late on Sunday afternoon I was helping with the preparations for supper. My right hip was now very stiff, forcing me to set my foot down in awkward positions each time I took a step. Actually I had very little control over where the foot went. The whole leg seemed to be stiffening: ankle, calf, knee. I moved around feeling as if I had a wooden appendage in tow. It began to dawn on me very slowly: the leg had the most peculiar sensation of numbness, but, my God, there was no pain as such. Also the pain in my back had disappeared completely. The spine moved easily and normally. I looked at my dinner in a state of wild exhilaration: for the first time in eighteen months, after I had taken 3 000 mg of Tegretol in twenty-six hours, the pain had faded.

My good luck held the following day. The back was normal, and the leg wooden but relatively pain-free. At 2.15 on Monday afternoon I phoned Green. I could not identify the woman at the other end of the line, but it was neither of the two I had spoken to on previous occasions.

"Good afternoon. This is Mrs. Birrer. May I have a word with Dr. Green, please?"

The voice at the other end gave a perceptible start. "Is that Mrs. Cynthia Birrer?"

"Yes."

"I am so sorry, Mrs. Birrer, but you cannot speak to him now."

"I insist on speaking to Dr. Green, right now."

"Please hold on." I heard the connection between her phone and his being made. A minute or so passed. "I am sorry, Mrs. Birrer, I cannot put you through."

"Please check once more. I want to make quite sure that Dr. Green will not speak to me."

The intercom clicked again. "I am so sorry, Mrs. Birrer, but he really is very busy."

"Fine. But please ask Dr. Green to phone me back when he is free. Tell him that I wish to discuss the regulation of my Tegretol dosage."

"Your Tegretol dosage?"

"Yes. Have you got that?"

"Yes, Mrs. Birrer, I'll see that he gets your message."

"Thank you."

I stared at the phone. Twenty-four hours seemed a reasonable time to wait for a busy doctor to return a phone call. However, by 6 p.m. on Tuesday Green had not yet phoned me back. I had mixed feelings. A tinge of sadness, perhaps, and deep disappointment. I knew that he had a fine brain; but there was no other force at work to transform this glorious gift into a healing instrument that could sustain the well-being of this patient, and maybe others. I had been abandoned by an intelligence that seemed to have been disciplined only by the infinite intricacies of the highly formalised training of a complex medical specialism. Undoubtedly these had been skilfully mastered, and he obviously took overweening pride in his accomplishment. But sometimes pride goes before a fall.

I pondered the question of a medical training: that is probably where a large part of the problem of technological barbarism in medical practice lies. In so many cases the men and women who enter our universities in order to make one of mankind's oldest and most revered professions their own are superbly trained; but they are not educated.

Dr. Szent-Gyorgyi, the eminent biomedical scientist, gets to the nub of the matter: "Desire to alleviate suffering is of small value in research - such a person should be advised to work for a charity. Research wants egoists, damn egoists, who seek their own pleasure and satisfaction, but find it in solving the puzzles of nature."[1]

It is, moreover, a dangerous quirk of human nature that it is often the most intelligent who are the least susceptible to being educated. And a superior intelligence that is not tempered by the humanitarian values that are the heritage of our civilisation spells disaster. This is never truer than in the case of those who take care of the sick. That the humanitarian element so often seems to be lacking in the medical personality makes one wonder whether the study of medicine should not be a post-graduate undertaking, and be preceded by adequate exposure to some form of liberal arts curriculum. In general, though, wisdom is the rich reward of a long life well lived,

1. Szent-Gyorgyi. Quoted in Katz, J.: *Experimentation with Human Beings.* New York, Russell Sage, 1973, p. 225.

and although it is not the prerogative of the old, it is very difficult indeed to inculcate it in the young. How do you put an old, or at least an experienced, head on young shoulders?

There are, of course, some ways of setting youthful feet on better paths, one of the most respected being the traditional code of ethics of the medical profession. It is always disheartening when we fail in our attempts, but sometimes our ineptitude is downright dangerous. Havoc is wreaked in the lives of individuals and their families and on a larger, macrocosmic scale in society itself. The bankruptcy of our social institutions is ever more clearly reflected in the rapidly deteriorating quality of our personal lives and in the irrevocable movement towards universal anarchy as we, the human race, plummet thunderously towards self-annihilation.

16

On Wednesday, 26th November, we began to make arrangements to seek further medical advice in Cape Town. I had to get an impartial opinion from a specialist who had not been thoroughly prejudiced before I reached him. In the meanwhile, I phoned Dr. Rice and reported the effects of the Tegretol.

"That *is* interesting." He told me to hold the daily dosage at six (1 200 mg) and to phone him every other day. Once again I was forcibly struck by the vast gulf separating his attitude on patient care from Green's. Once, when I had complained to a close friend of Green's about the latter's seeming unconcern, I was told, icily, by the comrade-in-arms that he did not know what I meant. A few minutes later he protested lamely, because he did know *exactly* what I meant: "But he's so *busy*. He sees *nineteen patients a day*. I've looked at his book. I've *told* him it's impossible to handle so many patients." Nineteen patients a day, and heaven - or the receptionist - help the twentieth. I nearly choked.

First, a doctor's busy-ness is the last excuse on earth he can invoke for neglecting a patient. Secondly, while it is true that Green, as one of a handful of neurologists practising in Johannesburg, is busy, he knows naught of the stress that busy-ness of a different and more exhausting complexity places on the conscience and competence of men like Rice – though, God knows, there are not many of them around. There had never been one occasion of the countless since 13th August when I had not been able to contact Rice. Once I waited fifteen minutes: I was placed on a side-line, constantly kept in touch and finally put through. There had never been one occasion when I could not make an appointment within forty-eight hours, and although I stood in a waiting room crammed to capacity until after 6 p.m., I saw the doctor. And there had never been one occasion when he failed to make a house visit within three to four hours of a call, often white with tension and fatigue. I thought more than once that it would be a miracle if he made it through another month without a coronary. As another patient said later, about her experience of the disease we have in common, a sad history of neglect and derision by a neurosurgeon: "If it had not been for our family doctor, I would have gone bananas." I knew just how she felt.

I did as Rice bid during the fortnight before we left for the Cape. There were no untoward incidents, although I scratched holes in the skin of my legs attempting to relieve the itch that had now appeared; but there was relatively no pain in the leg, none at all in the back, and the edge had definitely been taken off the burning. I was able to wear silky trousers without undue discomfort, although not for long, because the waist band continued to irritate the spine.

We were put into contact with Dr. Bell by Professor Jansen of the University of Cape Town. Years before Professor Jansen had operated on me at a time when I was at the end of my tether, also as the result of illness and its gross mismanagement. A few months after I met Bill, which was shortly after my first marriage ended, I began to have recurrent bouts of vomiting throughout the day. At first these looked like ordinary bilious attacks, minus the biliousness and nausea. I kept some food down, but a great deal of it came up. Over one year the projectile vomiting increased in severity until I could not even retain a glass of water. In retrospect I think that when this happened in a cinema or restaurant or private home, it was more embarrassing than epilepsy could ever be, for both of us.

After a month or so I went to see a general practitioner, who assured me that I was very pregnant. I almost fainted. My periods were late, but as that was not unusual I had not given the matter a second thought. He took a urine specimen and two days later confirmed the diagnosis. I could not summon the courage to tell Bill myself. He was much older than I was, and a genuinely confirmed bachelor. I was also not sure that I wanted to marry again, at least not yet. A friend broke the news to him, and I have never been able to ask how he took it. But there was really nothing we could do but accept the fact with grace and make the best of a terrible mistake. It was not what either of us would have chosen then, but for me there was no alternative. I cannot condone abortion, unless the life of the mother, or the infant, is in jeopardy. It was too late, not only for tears but for anything at all. We shut tight our respective mouths, made arrangements for the wedding and firmly agreed to grin and bear it. It was the beginning of seventeen happy years together, and our loveless match has never shown the kind of strains we continually see in those unions which, we are assured, were made in heaven, perhaps because we never had to cope with the inevitable demise of the impossible ideal of romantic love. We have always felt free to pursue our own interests, even when these do not coincide, but we are happiest together.

We went to Durban for our honeymoon. On the second day there I began to menstruate, quite normally, albeit three and half months late. Under the circumstances, what do you do? Laugh? Cry? Get a divorce? Cut your throat? Cut the doctor's throat? Well, we decided just to carry on and see. It would have been a flawless month except for the fact that fewer and fewer of my meals stayed down.

We arrived home and I started working systematically through the medical roster. I refused to return to my first choice because I did not honestly think it could be premature menopause; the second one suspected cardiac problems, the third said spastic colon, and the fourth, an ulcer - definitely. The radiologist decreed me wilful and wicked because I could not keep enough barium meal down for him to be able to say what it was. (Later Jansen said the pictures he did manage to take - after slapping me across the face while I was imprisoned behind the screen - were perfectly adequate, and although the repeats in Cape Town had less gas, due to preparatory colonic irrigation, anyone who knew what he was looking at could tell from either set what the matter was.) In the end, of course, the doctors did agree - I was hopelessly and irretrievably neurotic.

Faced with a pathology they could not recognise, they used the meanest of psychological tricks. They prevailed on Bill, who prevailed on me, to see a psychiatrist. I did, and we whiled away many vacuous hours talking animatedly and in great detail about nothing.

He thought shock treatment might help the depression that was developing as a result of the doctors' total inability to stop my vomiting, though it goes without saying that that was not the explanation he offered. Having no idea at all of what he was proposing, I agreed. The actual treatment itself and the concomitant amnesia, which I do not believe ever cleared completely, was a bitter experience. Never again was I able to glance at the page of a book for a few seconds and then reproduce it without error. But the hospital – I was an inmate – was set in rather lovely grounds, and as I walked endlessly around, always conscious of the blur of the green grass against the blue sky, since there was an English immigrant who railed incessantly against both, I thought of the ways there must be to deal with mental disorders. What was going on in that hospital did not appear to represent any significant advance on the snake pit. When I could stand it no longer and insisted on discharge, at least I came away with a clear notion of what I wanted to do. My first marriage had given me an unquenchable motivation to study; my painful clash with psychiatry had determined what it was I should study. I planned to make a career in psychology – but first I had to stop vomiting.

I asked for referral to a specialist in Cape Town and was sent to Dr. Werner. He examined me and then the X-rays and wrote out a prescription. It did not work. He tried again and that did not work either. He made several further attempts before he, too, climbed on the psychological band-wagon.

"Your wife is neurotic," he said to Bill, with an air that brooked no argument.

"No, my wife is not neurotic. My wife is sick. S-I-C-K." Bill stood up and slammed his fist on the desk. "There is a mechanical defect of some sort or another – you don't have to be a doctor to see that. I want every bloody X-ray retaken and I want the best man in Cape Town to do it."

Werner lifted his eyebrows. "Mr. Birrer, you are an architect – why don't you stick to reinforced concrete? But it is your money, I suppose. I'll speak to Dr. Drury."

Two days later, at 9 a.m., I was the first patient in Drury's surgery. He diagnosed a pyloric stenosis and phoned Werner before he took the first X-ray. I went back to Werner immediately afterwards with the plates. I shall never forget our meeting. He came around his desk, a faintly foreign-looking, short, slight man, excited, face wreathed in smiles. He put his arm around me and hugged me. He stepped between Bill and me, slipping one arm through mine, the other through Bill's.

"My dear, my dear, I made a mistake. I am so sorry, but I am so glad that we are going to be able to help you. We have just the man for the job here."

If I had a tape-recording of the occasion I would lodge it in the Museum of Medical Memorabilia. Such an event must surely be unique in the long history of the profession. A survey conducted in the United States revealed that many patients would never have sued their doctors but for the doctors' indifference when things in fact did go awry, and for their refusal to admit their faults. But doctors do not admit to mistakes, never mind apologise for them. Why should they? Either they can bury them, or they can flee from them to the safe haven of the fraternal bosom. Today the medical profession is so powerful that its members, free from any fear of public reprisal, grow ever more insensitive and unresponsive to the needs and the interests and the rights of the patient. Dead men tell no tales, and neither does any doctor: I'm OK., and he's O.K., and the devil take the patient. But at least I have met one doctor who knew when he was wrong, and said he was wrong, and acted to set the record straight. He came to see me on the day I was discharged from Groote Schuur Hospital and pumped my arm in unconcealed glee. "Look at you, just look at you, you are well, I am so glad, you are well." I am sorry I did not realise then how mighty was the gesture that he made, because he died shortly afterwards.

Yes, I was well when I left that hospital, and I remained fighting fit and brimful of energy for over ten years – running, never walking, often working eighteen hours a day without any feeling of strain. I had a career to carve out, I was in my mid-twenties, and there was a long way to go. I had no time to waste.

After our first meeting with Professor Jansen Bill and I agreed that it had not taken five minutes before it was as clear as daylight that this man could be trusted absolutely. Calm, competent, supremely confident, but without a trace of conceit. His eyes never left my face as I unfolded my story. I told how bitterly I resented the electro-shock treatments – each and every one of them; I regarded the therapy as a brutal and unwarranted violation of my integrity of mind, and it is one of the few things that I can never forgive. Jansen leaned towards me.

87

"But that is all over now. You are going to be better - quite, quite better. You are not going to be sick any longer."

He performed a Ladd's procedure, a surgical remediation of the pyloric stenosis that does not involve short-circuiting the bowel. The operation went like clockwork, and so did my rapid recovery. I received superlative care from the hospital staff, and morning and evening Jansen came in, patted my hand, chatted, joked, laughed, stole my sweets, brown eyes twinkling behind his spectacles - missing nary a thing, from the slight trace of huskiness in my throat, caused by the tube, to the temperature of my toes.

Professor Jansen runs a tight ship and there are no weak links in the moorings. I have never in my life, before or since, felt so safe, and I adored the man who guaranteed my security with his ceaseless and unwavering vigilance.

17

Promptly at 1 p.m. on 10th December, 1975, Dr. Bell came out to greet us in the ante-room of his surgery and ushered us into his inner sanctum. It was dull; the curtains were drawn across the wide windows. But I did not feel gloomy, then or later. In fact, I did not feel very much at all. Perhaps this *was* just another of that multitude of opinions Green snidely foresaw I would have to pry out somewhere. As my eyes grew accustomed to the diminished light I thought, no, maybe this time it was going to be all right. The face had the deep, comforting furrows of experience, the eyes shone kindly, and though the voice was tired, it reassured me.

He picked up his pen and I watched his hand move across the index card as, very soberly, he began to take down the details of the case. I tried hard to get the sequence of events correct and to duplicate as nearly as possible what I had told Kenny. Like Kenny, he often looked at me sharply; but his face was more mobile than Kenny's, and once or twice I thought I saw a flash of astonishment. I listened carefully to the story I was telling: a doctor's Agatha Christie. No wonder no one had been able to paint a picture that included all the details.

Bell asked many of the questions that Kenny had had on his list, but he also had a few of his own. He wanted to know why I thought I was having difficulty with my speech – was it just a question of finding the right word? No, that was not the problem; even when it did happen I could usually find a substitute without a perceptible pause. But I had a lazy eyelid; maybe I had a lazy tongue as well. It just lolled sluggishly on the floor of my mouth and I simply could not get it around words. I remembered when the first prolonged breakdown in my speech occurred. The words had stumbled out, slurred, contracted, incomprehensible. I had heard the gibberish with a mixture of horror and amazement and tried valiantly to get one sentence out straight. None came, just one unintelligible word after another. Nothing I said made sense. The pitch of my voice rose. The greater the effort, the poorer the result. My shoulders had become involved in it. I had felt my body tense. Leaning forward slightly, my fore-arms bent up, rigid, the knuckles of my hands so taut that they ached afterwards, I had felt my trunk begin to move first to the left and then to the right as if to force the words out. My hair had felt damp. I struggled for over twenty minutes before I broke down, completely unnerved.

As Bell moved from the top of my head to the soles of my feet he probed things I had been conscious of for the previous two to two and a half years, but which had not been considered by the other doctors. He wanted to know what my thought processes "felt" like. It took me some time before I found the word "compressed", and that was not very apt. Having a "head explosion" is one thing, readily identifiable and amenable to description. An angiogram, for example, is experienced as a series – about four in my case, I think – of head explosions, attenuated by the effects of the anaesthetic, which cannot be held completely at bay, although I had learnt, deliberately, to resist all but the largest doses during the shock treatment. But the experience of being crowded out of your body, squeezed aside, by your own thoughts turned in upon themselves is not something that I really felt I wanted to talk about – or could, for that matter.

In the short period since the diagnosis.of my condition I have given some thought to the psychology of the disease. Apart from the erosion of emotional life, the thinking process, which I believe generally remains intact throughout, plays some peculiar tricks, and there are times when mental activities proceed at a rate that is thoroughly exhausting. They are so lucid and vivid, they constitute very real noise. But the din does not *displace* words, thoughts; it *is* the ideas which chase each other around, interminably around, eventually crashing tumultuously into an unseen barrier, piling up, high, high, high, one on top of the other, pressing down hard when they reach their bony limits: thoughts demanding to be expressed. They spill over into the motor system, but the tongue refuses to convey them and the legs cannot run from them. The mind does not lack clarity, it is not tormented by formless images; it is not beset by vague fears. But the coherence beats hopelessly against the massive force of inertia. It seems to me that this tragic dilemma, more than anything else, holds the seeds of the final act of self-destruction, for as the disease progresses it must become virtually synonymous with the abolition of the spirit that powers the intention to act, while leaving the ability to form the intent inviolate. It is one of the more diabolical twists of fate. My safety valve is writing, since my right arm is only slightly affected; the hand cannot exceed a certain rate and the mind is bridled by it, providing some degree of volitional control over thinking.

Bell's examination was very similar to those conducted by both Green and Kenny. In addition he examined the skin on the forehead for evidence of more profuse sweating on one side than on the other. He found this on the right, and I gathered that he was satisfied that the constricted pupil was Horner's syndrome. Later in the examination he attempted to elicit abdominal reflexes. These were present. His face, tautening as he worked over the legs and hips for more than ten minutes, relaxed. "Good, good," he muttered.

He measured my thighs carefully in three different places with a tape; they were identical He applied the twin points of a compass at several levels along the inner surface of the right arm above the wrist. Regardless of the distance between the compass points, I could not distinguish them. Nor was there any sensation of the vibrations in the small circular base of a large tuning fork when this was applied to joints of the limbs on the right side. I told him that I still experienced hearing loss periodically on the left, as well as the right, and he spent minutes testing both ears. He put the middle finger of his right hand behind my left lobe and pushed it gently upwards.

"The nerve has gone."

While I dressed he moved into an adjoining room with the X-rays. He came back twelve minutes later. He did not agree that there was a Chiari. "Whatever you call it, it is not causing your problems." By now, those sounds were familiar. We both sat down and I waited while he wrote up his findings. When he looked up Bill asked him if he had reached any conclusion. He raised both hands a few inches above the desk, placed the tips of his fingers together and leaned forward. I don't think he enjoyed the next few minutes very much.

"The burning you are experiencing in your lower back and legs is due to a condition known as arachnoiditis. It is a rare and dreaded reaction to a myelogram. It makes one wonder whether myelograms ought to be done, particularly when a patient is as severely affected as you are." Arachnoiditis is the inflammation, or scarring, of one of the three meninges, or coverings of the spinal cord. "You ought to have hydrocortisone in the spine – three shots should be enough. But even so it will be a few months before it subsides. Without it, the painful burn will continue indefinitely. If you were my patient, you would have the first shot today. Has no one suggested cortisone?"

"In absolute desperation I asked for the stuff. It was refused."

I recalled the unctuous proclamation of cortisone as an assault on the system. A great moralist, is Green. I wondered what the hell he thinks unsupervised dosages of Tegretol are? Or a myelogram, God help me, where due precautions against health hazards have not been taken? Or the firm recommendation for a discogram on a lumbar disc that the radiologist's report asserts is sound?

I'd managed to get out of the discogram, at any rate. I felt detached, a childlike sense of wonder. What am I, a masochist or something? They had trapped me before, these doctors, twice, and here I was once again, older but just as stupid, and now the results were not merely a passing touch of amnesia. Sure, there were no headaches, no fever, following that Tuesday in January when the myelogram was done, just the seeds of crippling spinal adhesions, insidious, debilitating internal injury. I hadn't tumbled to it, but someone else had. Jill's face, framed by the burnished jet hair, slipped in and out of focus. Her quiet, measured tones repeated over and over again: "Cynthia, that dye, the Myodil . . .?" Questioning, insisting, pleading – but never heeded. What about the Myodil? Surely the medical maestro that I had taken such pains to find would know what to do about the Myodil?

I forced my head to empty, felt my throat parch, conscious in every fibre that there was worse to come, if that was possible.

Bell glanced downwards, and leaned back.

"The more critical question, however, concerns the nature of the problems that caused you to have the myelogram in the first place."

I thought the wrinkling at the corner of his eyes increased, just a little. There was no need for either of us to speak. He leaned forward again, fingertips now pressed tightly together.

"Mrs. Birrer, you have consulted other specialists and my opinion carries no more weight, but no less, than theirs. This is an exceedingly complex clinical picture. However, it is my opinion that you have multiple sclerosis."

I looked at him. Maybe he was wrong.

He looked at me. "Maybe I'm wrong. When you get back to Johannesburg I want you to see Dr. Evans. He has taken a special interest in this disease for a number of years. He can confirm the diagnosis. Maybe he can also help you."

Multiple sclerosis is a disease of the central nervous system which follows no set pattern. Its onset is often accompanied by impaired vision and stumbling due to affected balance. In some cases the sufferer may even be blind and paralysed at the outset but recover and never have another symptom for the rest of his life. It is now believed that these symptoms are caused by a virus which has a short (24-36 hour) period of infectivity attacking the white matter of the brain and spinal cord. This strips the myelin, or insulating sheath, off the nerve fibres. The nervous system symptoms may become manifest only about fifteen to twenty years later, when the degeneration, or demyelinating process, prevents messages from reaching the brain, thereby resulting in a loss of senses, such as touch.

The disease usually follows a course of relapses and remissions which can vary enormously in frequency. Remissions occur when the body's natural resources repair the damage, but "it tends to be a botched affair – rather like a bad electrical connection", [1] and there is always a possibility of relapse. Scientists at the Institute for Research on Mental Retardation, Staten Island, New York, and at the University of Philadelphia's School of Medicine are working on a vaccine that will prevent the disease. They are also searching for some means of stimulating resistance in people already suffering

1. Currie, S.: *The Yorkshire Post News Service*, 27 January, 1976.

from it.

One of the more interesting aspects of multiple sclerosis is that it has for more than thirty years been known to have a geographical distribution. The general rule of thumb for its incidence is that the further a country is situated away from the equator, the greater the chance is of its inhabitants contracting the disease. The disorder is most common in Ireland, and is also seen in the United Kingdom, Europe and the United States. In Southern Africa it is known among whites, though it occurs much less commonly among those born here. At the busy neurology department of Baragwanath Hospital for Africans in Johannesburg there is no single case of multiple sclerosis on record. Three suspected cases have been seen in Kenyans and in a young African man from Rhodesia who went to study in the United States. Dr. Evans suspects that I myself contracted multiple sclerosis during an extended period of study in Philadelphia, when for nearly two years I could not shake off persistent bronchitis. However, in no cases involving Africans has the diagnosis ever been definitely established.

We spoke about the disease in general terms for a while longer. Well over an hour had passed when we rose to go. We thanked Dr. Bell sincerely for the great effort he had so clearly expended. We respected his integrity, recognising that there was an emotional price not only for ourselves, but for him as well. In this instance, a job well done had a pretty rotten return.

18

When I saw Bell on that Wednesday, 10th December, I was feeling a little disturbed about the events of the previous two days, but as I thought they would pass I did not mention them to him. It had struck me on that Monday that I was urinating rather frequently – every ten to fifteen minutes. But that was not as alarming as the speed with which the floor seemed to swirl up to meet me when I bent my head forward to rise from the toilet seat. The first time it happened, just before morning tea, I snapped my head back and rashly tried to stand up. I involuntarily lifted my arms to the level of my shoulders on each side, just touching the walls on both sides with my finger tips. The edge of the seat, pressed against the inner surface of both legs in the region of the knees, forced me to lean backwards. The back of my head struck the wall. The next second, with an awful clatter of seat against pan, I literally hurtled into the right-hand wall. The hand basin pushed into my waist somewhere on the left. I tried to steady myself with the left arm, but instead spun through one hundred and eighty degrees, veered backwards and lost my balance completely, smashing into the door with the back of my head and shoulders. As I slid down, dazed, my left leg shot upward, sharply catching the outer edge of the seat; it flew up noisily. Time passed, but I stayed where I was, head slumped forward, eyes closed, waiting until this crazy world righted itself. Then I strained upward, clutched the edge of the hand basin with my left, pressed against the rim of the pan as well as I could with a numbed right hand, and somehow got onto my feet. My head ached. After a while I risked opening the door. Thank goodness we were staying with friends. I made it to the couch in the sitting room. Within twenty-four hours the inner calf of the left leg, from knee to ankle, was a lurid shade of purple.

During the week that followed these attacks occurred, though in a milder form, each time I went to the lavatory - which was often. However, I invented a technique of getting through the procedure without ever actually falling again, although I did reel dizzily on one or two occasions. But on the Thursday events took a nasty turn. Now I began to lose my balance whenever I looked downward to check where I was putting my feet. I decided to move around as little as possible, and spent most of my time on the couch in my gown. I tried to get dressed, but there was so much bending involved that I gave it up, hoping the spells would pass.

Late Saturday afternoon I was treading my way carefully to the kitchen to make a few snacks. I remember beginning to lose my balance, and beginning to run, trying to get somewhere, anywhere, before I fell. My next recollection was a feeling of wetness on my face and a bursting throb in my mouth. I drew my hand gingerly across my mouth and glanced at it. It was covered in blood. I thought in a dull sort of way that a tooth must have been knocked out - my crowning glory, Bill once called my teeth. Fortunately it was only my nose, the bridge battered by its contact with the arm of an upholstered chair which had prevented me from hurtling through a large, paneless window into space and a concrete slab three floors below.

I was put onto a bed, and one ice pack after another was applied to my sore face to counteract the bruising. Left alone briefly while the other three ate dinner, I got up with the intention of changing into pyjamas. I made towards the bathroom with that thought in my mind.

When I came round a large, corpulent form was looming over me. He noticed my open eyes.

"Mrs. Birrer, Mrs. Birrer. Can you hear me?"

I could, perfectly well. I could see him just as clearly. But I could not utter a sound.

"I am Dr. Kane. Your friends have asked me to look at you. You have hurt yourself." I noticed the needle in his hand, but slipped away again, momentarily. Then he asked if "it" hurt; I felt nothing, but a moment later there was a sharp jab.

"That hurt, you bastard." I passed out.

Later, the two pieces of my left ear firmly rejoined with seven stitches, I became interested enough to want to join the doctor and Bill in a cup of tea. Bill explained that we were due to return to Johannesburg the following day. The doctor's kindly face registered horror at the thought.

"She is not to leave that bed before Wednesday at the earliest."

I began to object, but passed out twice more instead.

I woke at about six the next morning; all I was aware of was a determination to return home that day. I had been thoroughly pampered during my stay, but I wanted my own bed, my own doctor. More than anything else, I wanted to see Evans and settle the matter. I walked slowly to the bathroom and did the minimum toileting necessary to make me nice to be near. Treading a perfectly straight line, I came back to the dressing table, rummaged around in my vanity case for any cosmetic to brighten those pallid cheeks, tone down that frightful greeny-yellow bruise covering my nose, lighten the deep, dark rings under both eyes and disguise the now hideously pronounced ptosis. I was considering my appearance with great distaste when something about my reflection caught my attention: horrified I watched the image split rapidly into two. My God, one was bad enough. Looking around the room and then through the window to the street, with the sea beyond, I found there was two of everything. It was my first attack of double vision since January. It could not have come at a more inconvenient time. I

95

looked, as Dr. Rice said the next day, as though I had been playing with Cassius Clay. And now, when I tried any repair work, my hand shot past my stitched ear. Well, I'd married an artist, so I called him over.

"Can you fix it? At least get my eyebrows on." Bill looked dubious. By the time he had finished, the sight in my right eye was so blurred I could not inspect the results.

The two men carried me into the car and at the airport a wheel chair transferred me to the plane. Approximately three and a half hours later I crept gratefully between the two cool sheets of my own bed.

The following day Dr. Rice called at the house. As I woefully recounted the events of my second abortive holiday, the tears rolled down my cheeks. I was stretched to the absolute limit; I did not know how much longer I could carry on, debilitated, in pain, and now very worried. Before he left, promising to get an appointment with Evans at the earliest opportunity, Dr. Rice prescribed tranquillisers, and this time I needed them.

The sister at his surgery phoned me the following day. An appointment had been made for Thursday, 18th December.

Again the endless story, the tests I had come to know so well (and now the double vision was back), the laborious commitment of details to paper. When Dr. Evans had finished we looked at each other for a long moment. It seemed like forever. I felt so tired. It really did not matter what he said.

"There is no possible alternative to the diagnosis of multiple sclerosis."

I pushed the hair back from my face with both hands.

"Can you do anything to arrest it?"

"I personally believe that the principal factor in the etiology of the disease is a virus which probably attacks the body in childhood, or at puberty. Since no one knows what the virus is, no one can cure multiple sclerosis. You know that. But I have a method of treatment which is not generally accepted by my colleagues. I believe that I have had some successes, but I have also had failures."

I could not really see what criteria could be used to determine success in the treatment of this disease, but I pushed my doubts into the back of my mind.

"You must understand I cannot offer any miracle cure. All I can do is try to stabilise the disease, but you *must* understand that it is no more than an experiment."

"What kind of treatment? How long?"

"To begin with, you will be in hospital for at least a month."

That meant virtually until the end of January. When would I be able to work again – after the Easter break?

"You cannot work for at least twelve months."

I gazed at the wall above Bill's head. I examined the ceiling in great detail without registering a single detail. I looked and looked, but I could not see. I remembered distantly that Keats had once said that there is no fiercer hell than the failure of a great ambition. The world began to spin a little. But suddenly, inexplicably, it stopped. It steadied. I chipped a bit of nail polish off my right thumbnail and made a mental note to do a bit more for my hands. Everything was all right. Nothing important had changed. I had earned inalienable membership in Academe: I was a student and I could continue to learn, and to teach. Nothing could stop that. True, there are rituals in the institutions within the world of learning, such as lecturing, in which perhaps I could no longer fully participate, but that was only a miniscule part of the enterprise, and not always a very rewarding one. I was a part of that esoteric universe, and my membership was direct; there was no need for mediation by any person or any body. If I chose, and if I was sufficiently independent intellectually – and the events of 1974 had made me so – I could continue to make a contribution until the day I died, which was as likely to be in a motor car accident as anything else. I recognised, of course, that certain limitations would be placed on my activities, but I would cross each bridge as I came to it. The point was that if I had to go it alone, I could do so.

Every intellectual lives in diaspora; to the extent he does not, he is barren. Furthermore, every intellectual has his own diaspora centre. For some, like Hemingway, it is humanity itself, so that self-exile in Paris, away from his native America, served only to sharpen his insight, deepen his understanding. In my own case it is the word, written or spoken. Where there are books, an assembly of the collective wisdom of human thought throughout the ages, life will continue to bear fruit. But even if I were isolated from the ideas of others, I carry within my own head all that I wish to possess. The impedimenta of contemporary life, the pretty clothes and baubles I loved in my teens, mean nothing. And neither do the impedimenta of my own

97

body, provided their destruction by disease does not hinder the effluence of mind.

All in all, however, I did not feel good when I left Dr. Evans. I still had to live out the grand theory. My brave new world was still somewhere in the future, and it was to take me about three weeks to make the adjustment to the knowledge that I had multiple sclerosis. Some time during each twenty-four hours in that period, the implications of what I might face hit me. My stomach would contract; my hair felt damp, as though I was running a temperature. Never a good sleeper, I found that sleep eluded me with a persistence Lady Macbeth could not have imagined. I knew it would pass, as everything under the sun passes, but it was hell at the time.

I was also extremely puzzled. Within the preceding month I had seen two neurologists and a neurosurgeon. Each had heard my sad tale in detail and conducted a meticulous examination. Comparing the three occasions, I could not really find any major differences. True, I had had the acute attack of vertigo, injuring myself twice, and the double vision and the blurring in the right eye had started again, and only Evans knew of this. But did these developments place a totally different light on the picture? They could not, because Bell had made his diagnosis without knowing about them. There were now two unequivocal diagnoses of multiple sclerosis. It therefore seemed very odd indeed that Kenny had "found nothing wrong with me". I made an appointment to see him on Wednesday, 24th December.

When we were settled Kenny asked whether anything had occurred since my previous visit. I told him about the vertigo, and that I had injured myself on two occasions. He noted it down.

"Mr. Kenny, I have been given two unequivocal diagnoses of multiple sclerosis."

He broke in: "From whom?"

"Bell in Cape Town and Evans here. Bell referred me back to Evans. I understand from Dr. Green that you could find nothing wrong with me. We would like to know what conclusions you actually reached."

"Green thinks there is a very large psychological overlay in your case. He believes that what cannot be accounted for by the Chiari is due to psychological factors. You are making mountains out of symptoms that are only molehills."

"Dr. Green thinks that I am hysterical, does he not?"

Kenny did not answer. "I know that he does, Mr. Kenny, because I have been told so by another doctor. It is also the inference I have made from things which he has said and done, and from the consultation I had with Professor Barron."

Kenny looked at me quietly. "Do you think your problems could be psychological?"

I returned Kenny's gaze. What I did think was that I might commit murder if I ever again heard another specialist, other than a psychiatrist (and I was not enamoured of them, either), utter that word. *Why* can doctors not confine themselves to the expert, *humane* practice of the skills they have taken so long to acquire, and for which the patient pays good money? They are generally uninformed regarding the fundamentals of the human and social aspects of biology. They are often palpably ignorant of contemporary psychology, and therefore of the emotional and cognitive components of human interaction. Moreover, if they do have any grasp at all of such things they constantly ignore the effects of psychobiological events as they occur in the lives of the patients and their families. I fail to see how else the continued refusals to speak to the husband of a patient can possibly be legitimately explained. Why must doctors always dabble in the ineffable? But psychology is their scapegoat, and they use it without compunction, anywhere, anytime.

I bit my tongue, feeling my anger subside. For the umpteenth time exhaustion began to steal over me. I sighed. It was a pity, really, that my problems were not psychological; I had one or two students who could do a better job than these boys had managed so far. Or I could do something about my own psyche. As it was, I was utterly dependent on the skill and humanism of a medical specialist who had some proficiency in the one area, and a serious deficiency in the other.

"No," I said, wearily. "I do not think that my problems could be psychological, Mr. Kenny."

He peered over the rim of his glasses at Bill. "Do you?"

"No," Bill echoed harshly, more angry than Kenny could possibly have known. "I do not. We have had this nonsense, and much more, with the medical profession before, here and in Rhodesia. We have been forced before to go elsewhere before anyone would recognise that my wife was sick."

Kenny tugged a typed report out of my pale blue file. "This is what I said about your case, Mrs. Birrer; my conclusions are at the end." He was distinctly displeased about something.

I took the typed pages. At the bottom of the third page, under the subtitle "Conclusions", two words, the very last two, leapt off the page: Multiple Sclerosis.

"Does this mean that you think that I have multiple sclerosis?"

"I think that you could very well have it. Let me check you over again."

He did so, working from his report and making pencilled notes on it. When he was finished, he seemed satisfied that what he found tallied with what he had written before. I sat on the edge of the couch, legs swinging gently, and expressed surprise at what Green thought about my case. Kenny left his instrument table and came over to me.

"What Green thinks about you as a person does not mean a thing in your life. I think a great deal of Bell, and Evans has been interested in multiple sclerosis for some years. They think you have the disease, and I do, too."

"Bell said it did not affect the length of life," I said irrelevantly.

"That is not the point. It radically affects the quality of life."

"Yes, I know that. Evans has some kind of treatment. I don't know what to do. What do you think?"

"You have no options. Bell can offer you nothing. As a surgeon, I can offer you nothing. Take the treatment and believe that it will help you."

He was frank. He was positive. But above all he understood my dilemma within the context of how I could cope, with the resources that I had at my disposal. I was looking at a doctor whom a patient could lean on when the going got tough, someone who could give just the right kind of support, in just the right quantity, at just the right moment.

On 29th December I was admitted to a Johannesburg clinic. The following day treatment to arrest the progress of an incurable disease began.

Part II Closed Shop

1

As I left Mr. Kenny after my second visit, l turned toward him: "I suppose that if you can think yourself *into* a disease, you can also . . . think yourself *out* of it." We finished the sentence in unison. I was touched by his calm sincerity, and we both smiled faintly.

Actually, I did not believe that I *could* think myself out of multiple sclerosis; what I did believe, very firmly, was that I could achieve a realistic acceptance of the disease, based on an understanding of it, and continue a full and productive life. It wasn't exactly easy, but I did discover an iron determination to pursue my research and writing and – though God only knows where it came from – the unshakable conviction that my best work lay in the future. I could have accepted the fact that I had multiple sclerosis without breast-beating and wailing, coming to terms with an incurable disease that was no longer an empty abstraction, and generally getting on with the business of living and working, had it not been for the complication of arachnoiditis. I had been told that the only means whereby this could be treated involved the introduction of a particular type of cortisone into the spine, a procedure Dr. Evans would not countenance in a patient with multiple sclerosis. This meant an indefinite period of pain and suffering, and there are times when it is still unbearable. This is especially so before and during menstruation, when deep, dragging agony binds body to bed for the simple reason that I do not have the strength in my legs to stand upright, although erect posture does afford a measure of relief. That I had arachnoiditis placed a different complexion altogether on the case.

I began to develop an inflammatory tertiary condition: psychosclerosis, which is Hardening of the Heart. The symptoms are the increasingly acute perception, after careful consideration of the sequence of bygone events, that one has been Buggered About. The effects are a dis-ease of sometimes appalling severity. This time, at least, it was clear that the problem was not psychological: I was stricken by a Real burn in a Real leg from a Real myelogram that may not Really have been necessary, but that had certainly been Really neglected. The question was: what ought to be done about it. I decided to sue Green.

In comtemporary society the medical practitioner is, more than ever before, deeply involved with the law. Professor S.A. Strauss of the University of South Africa has observed that in this country there is no profession whose conduct is more comprehensively regulated by law than that of the physician. From the legal point of view, the medical profession has become one of the most hazardous of all. "The practice of medicine is pregnant with the potentiality of lawsuits by patients against physicians."[1] Casual examination of the cases reported in South Africa during the past fifty years or so reflects the extent to which doctors have been harassed by malpractice actions, both founded and unfounded. It is possible to cite an impressive list of professional errors which ultimately led to verdicts against medical defendants. To mention only a few: superficial examination of the patient leading to a wrong diagnosis; premature operation; failure to refer the patient to a specialist; use of wrong or outdated technique; wrong prescription; excessive dosage; abandonment of the patient; failure to instruct the patient properly. Hardly a month passes without a report in the press of some actual or potential action against a doctor. Nevertheless, the medical practitioner has in general received "soft" treatment at the hands of the law. In the majority of cases involving malpractice litigation, the doctor is exonerated. In some of the early cases reported during the nineteenth century where the decision went against the doctor, the judges were almost apologetic for handing down an adverse decision. Strauss conjectures that there must have been so few medical practitioners in colonial days that judges were reluctant to discourage them through an adverse judgment against one of them.

I approached my attorney, a partner in a leading legal firm in Johannesburg. The major stumbling block to the pursuit of justice in a case where the patient believes suffering has been incurred due to the indifference and poor judgment of a specialist was immediately obvious. If the lawyer is to serve the plaintiff well, the case must be formulated so that there is at least a reasonable chance of success

1. Strauss, S.A.: "The legal remedy which is a medical nightmare". *Codicillus,* 8, 1966.

in a court of law. To do less places the plaintiff in danger of incurring thousands of rands in legal costs if he loses the case. On the other hand, if a doctor loses he is unlikely to suffer severe financial losses, since most members of the medical profession are insured against this possibility. To all intents, the real defendant is not so much the doctor himself as his insurance company – "a slick and dehumanised corporation of steel and concrete with millions",[1] as Dr. Klass calls it.

Unfortunately, few legal men, if any, possess the medical knowledge necessary to formulate a substantial case where this depends upon a wide grasp of the intricate facts of the disease and the medical procedures in question. They are therefore dependent upon the co-operation of a member, or members, of the medical profession in the capacity of an expert witness. This is no more than an expression of the fundamental principle of the adversary trial system, namely that it is for the parties to lay evidence before the court and that the court will never take the initiative in investigating the facts at issue. The parties must therefore call witnesses, whether laymen or experts, and the court may not, of its own accord, call any witness. However, it is extremely difficult, and sometimes impossible, to find an expert medical witness to testify for the prospective plaintiff. Dr. Evans, who several times expressed the view that I was "a victim of *malicious* negligence", refused – on the three occasions when I pleaded and remonstrated with him – to speak to my attorney in connection with the case. I made one such request after he had witnessed a spell of violent pain in the evening of the day on which the Tegretol was discontinued. Only Tegretol and Pethidine afforded me any relief from the pain, but Evans stopped the former when it seemed that the toxic side-effects of the heavy dosages were aggravating respiratory depression.

Dr. Evans saw the extent and degree of my suffering and it worried him deeply. He deplored Green's conduct and his handling of the case in the strongest possible terms, both to me and to my husband separately, and also when we were together. But, like others, he was not willing to co-operate with my lawyer in the vital preliminary stages of the preparation of a case against Green. Obviously, such refusals are a real impediment, because the burden of prov-

1. A. Klass. Quoted in Strauss, S.A.: "Medical negligence. In Doctor & Law". *Documenta Geigy*, 4, 1969, p. 4.

ing his case upon a balance of probability rests on the plaintiff.

It is difficult to escape the impression, when canvassing expert testimony, that side by side with some astonishing advances in medical science, the fraternity has developed an inverted genius that may betoken a significant increase in average life expectancy coupled with a significant decrease in concern for the over-all quality of that life. I really felt I had slipped through the looking glass when I listened to a top radiologist, aided by a standard text on myelography and a ruler, lucidly set out the criterial attributes of a certain anomaly of the hindbrain and then go on to demonstrate beyond all doubt why the protrusion in the picture of my own skull did not meet those criteria - *and yet knew* that the expert would not, and the textbook could not, be brought into court as testimony in an allegation of mistaken, and negligently mistaken, identity. The profession apparently has developed a Medea-like intensity to paralyse conscience, and a steady erosion of both human values and humane consideration for the patient has clearly taken place during the different phases of the industrial revolution.

Once legal proceedings are under way, of course, any number of physicians may be subpoenaed as expert witnesses in the hope of obtaining a favourable opinion. The legal right possessed by a party to a suit is to subpoena the medical witness to attend court and then to ask him questions relevant to the particular matter at issue, which the practitioner must answer if ordered to do so by the court. Apart from the glaring weakness of this approach, the old adage of leading a horse to water applies, despite the fact that failure to obey a subpoena without lawful excuse constitutes contempt of court. Moreover, the plaintiff and his counsel are always conscious that the case may simply explode in the face of medical facts of which they were either not fully cognizant or which have not been appropriately presented. Lawyers, and this plaintiff, accept as a matter of course that their opponents shall question and challenge their position at every turn in litigation, because it is only by searching inquiry that the truth is established. It therefore behooves both parties to be prepared for every contingency.

Yet, as the situation presently exists, very few doctors will assist an attorney in such matters. Only rarely will a doctor comment on the behaviour of a colleague or on his conduct of a case. The medical fraternity closes its ranks, and these remain tightly shut no matter how justified any member may quite obviously feel your cause to be. I think, somewhat wryly, that these men are unbelievably noble in denying that one of their number may have been unconscionably delinquent when astonishment and disbelief is written in every line of their faces on their being confronted with the facts of the case, and when they are able completely to demolish a diagnosis (off the record, of course) on what appear to be impeccable grounds.

The situation is patently incongruous. When a person in a so-called democratic society believes – rightly or wrongly – that an injustice has been perpetrated, the matter can, and should, be debated in a court of law. Arising out of centuries of experience, a system of jurisprudence has evolved under which, through the vigorous contest between the parties to the case, we seek to establish the truth. Where a decision is reached that is unacceptable to either side, the machinery exists for further action to be taken. However, this is a costly procedure and no responsible lawyer will advise a client to go ahead with it unless he feels there is a reasonable chance of winning the case. For those who do not have unlimited financial resources this very large element of chance in seeking redress for alleged malpractice by a doctor effectively closes the orthodox arena of justice. It is an anomaly that must be set right. No man should, in effect if not in principle, be beyond the reach of the law, for whatever reason. In this decade we have ample evidence that not even the president of the most powerful country in the West is exempt from democratic justice.

2

The basis of the professional liability of a physician is fault in the form of the delict of negligence. Delict is the Roman-Dutch synonym of the Anglo-American term "tort". "In strict legal analysis negligence means more than heedless or careless conduct, whether in omission or commission: it properly connotes the complex of duty, breach and damage thereby suffered by the person to whom the duty was owing."[1] A delict is conduct by a person that con-

1. Nathan, H. L.: *Medical Negligence: Legal Case Studies.* London, Butterworth, 1957, p. 2.

stitutes a civil wrong and that renders the perpetrator liable under law to pay pecuniary damages to the injured party. The law of delict is largely personal injury law. The dramatis personae in almost any personal injury case are constant: the plaintiff, the court and the defendant - another name for what is, quite often, an insurance company.

Among the delicts that are embodied in the scope of medical professional liability are assault (intentional violation of personal integrity), fraud, defamation and *iniuria* in the form of a breach of confidential, personal communications or a violation of privacy.

With regard to the violation of personal integrity, at no time while he was handling my case, or later, on careful reflection in tranquillity, did I impute malice to any of Green's actions. Whatever else Green is answerable for, I personally found no malice. Whether there is an element of *professional* malice that served to militate against referral is another story altogether.

The claim is liability for negligence, and where such an allegation is made only another doctor, or panel of doctors, can assess whether the plaintiff has a *prima facie* case, and advise an attorney accordingly. By decree of the courts in South Africa medical negligence is, to a large extent, determined by the standards of reasonable care set by the doctors themselves. But a doctor is the very last person who will speak out on these matters, and his refusal to do so undermines the legal process, which rests upon expert testimony, thereby tearing at and mutilating the warp and woof of the social fabric. Surely there is a point at which a doctor must acknowledge that allegiance to humanity itself supersedes the code that binds him to his professional brother? And surely there is a point at which he must be prepared to act on this resolve for the sake of the greater good?

The decision to do so depends upon a form of professional and individual responsibility that places loyalty to fellow men above that to a colleague guilty of illegal or negligent activity. Obviously this attitude is open to abuse, but that has long been considered an acceptable risk of free speech, within very broad limits. But what is far more important is that this danger can scarcely exceed the threat to the patient that inheres in the doctor's failure to meet his contractual obligations, or to observe the highest ethics of his profession. The last line of defence that a patient has, against the denial of his rights by his doctor's betrayal of trust and abuse of power, is the willingness and ability of responsible members of the medical fraternity to co-operate in formulating a case that may be placed before the courts, and to offer apposite testimony before a judge when this has been done.

From where comes the code that makes every doctor his brother's keeper? For the layman, the question is difficult to answer. Probably it is caught rather than taught during the long rigorous years of a medical training. Most of medical education takes place in tightly knit, conforming groups. As a result, the majority accept the general ideas about society that are set by the conventional wisdom of their peers. It is not by accident, but rather by training and conditioning, that most doctors are conservative and anti-radical in their views. Clinical training is by precept and not debate; "yes, sir" is the name of the ward-rounds game. Non-conformity in any area of thought is shunned and becomes subject to subtle, covert sanctions, unofficial but powerful enough to make most doctors fall in line, and to keep them beholden one to another.

Melvin M. Belli, who originally won fame in the United States as the King of Torts, characterises its effect as the "conspiracy of silence" amongst medical men, "the silent medical treatment", the reluctance – nay, the refusal – of physicians to testify against defendant brethren. However, to implicate all medical men as cold-blooded members of an esoteric brotherhood, deliberately pledged to silence for their mutual benefit, without the slightest regard for the interests of the patient who suffers through lack of skill or through inadvertence on the part of his doctors, is crass and facile.

It is true that medicine was originally magic, and although doctors do sometimes seem to be little more than a close-knit band of sorcerers, the critical factor in this last quarter of the twentieth century is the staggering impact that the spirit of industrialism has had on ethical relations in every sphere of contemporary life, from sexual relationships to medical practice. During the nineteenth century the physician became more and more impersonal, more of a businessman and less influenced by the social and ethical obligations that were a characteristic of the eighteenth-century physician. The family doctor of yester-year has well-nigh disappeared, except in small communities, and idealism everywhere is yielding to the material ideal of clean-cut business efficiency. It is to the credit of modern medicine that despite intense competition the majority of doctors have continued to practice their profession along time-honoured lines, although it is a truism that in the money markets of the world a man whose heart is better than his head is a fool by definition.

The almost insuperable barrier which keeps the doctor from business-like efficiency and its financial rewards, and at the same time encourages him to adopt any stratagem that will help him to avoid the inevitable liabilities of commercial inefficiency, particularly in the post-Nader era, is the fact that whether he has a speciality or not, the doctor's task is one of arduous complexity. The practice of medicine is not an exact science, and the doctor's margin of error is very small indeed – "the margin between safety and danger sometimes measures little more than the thickness of a sheet of paper". [1] This is probably truer in the case of the nervous system than in that of any other part of the body. We are light years away from a complete understanding of the brain and its functioning – if this is indeed possible, involving as it does a logical paradox – and it may well be deemed a miracle that neurologists, and their professional kissing-cousins the neurosurgeons, have come as far as they have in the treatment of disorders of the central nervous system. No matter how fine the neurologist's own brain is, he is beset by pitfalls at every turn, and he may even be justified in claiming some additional immunity from the wrath of a patient for bona fide errors. And I think that it must be accepted that, no matter how unfortunate the consequences are for the patient – even the occurrence of a rare and unexpected complication, or of death itself – doctors are human, they are not infallible and they can and do make bona fide errors, for which they should not be crucified.

It is absolutely mandatory in malpractice litigation to strike a reasoned balance between the protection of the legitimate interests of a patient injured through medical negligence, and protection for the medical profession in its service to mankind. If this is not established there may be various consequences, the most serious of all being that the ever-present fear of possible legal action might inhibit medical practitioners in rendering assistance to the public. Thus, as Strauss has observed, doctors might tend to avoid procedures which, although valuable, carry great risk for certain individuals. A myelogram, of course, falls into this category: it has an inherent ele-

1. Stetler, J. and Moritz, A. R.: *Doctor and Patient and the Law.* St. Louis, Mosby Co., 1971.

ment of risk, against which due precaution must be taken if performing it is unavoidable through lack of a more benign substitute. But there can be no question of stopping the use of successful drugs or of discontinuing useful procedures because individual idiosyncrasy exists and has been statistically charted.

Every biologist knows that within a group of living organisms there is always an individual variation in the sensitivity to a poison or a drug. Because of natural biological variation some individuals are affected more than others, and some may not be affected at all. If about 0,5 mg of strychnine is given by intraperitoneal injection to a certain strain of rats, approximately 50% of the animals die. But the fact that the other 50% survive cannot be taken as evidence against a causal relation between the intake of strychnine and death in rats.

The unavoidable fact of individual variation which the doctor falls back on as the ultimate justification for an untoward result, explaining it at great length with punctilious patience, places him squarely upon the horns of a dilemma that he simply does not seem to comprehend. Precisely because differences among people do exist, and precisely because an outcome in a given patient *cannot* be predicted with certainty, *any* "therapeutic" intervention (or non-intervention) is "experimental". To put it more concretely: expert witnesses before the Senate Sub-committee on Health in America recently disagreed about whether psychosurgery - that is, brain surgery for the purpose of modifying behaviour - is in fact therapeutic.

Until recently - that is, until roughly the last half-century - clinical investigation involving the use of human subjects was closely tied to therapeutic procedures in medicine. When physicians employed new drugs, or surgeons utilised new and previously untried procedures in the treatment of patients, public concern was at a minimum, principally because it was virtually impossible to distinguish between the prerogatives of the physician in exercising professional judgment in respect of which method of treatment should be recommended.

There is a large grey area of uncertainty as to what is medical treatment and what is medical investigation. In fact, any therapeutic procedure is an experiment in any individual case, because no two persons, except single-ovum twins, are genetically identical. This is true whether the specialist acknowledges the procedure as experimental or not. Obviously a doctor who exalts clinical medicine, as does Green, tacitly makes this admission. Any therapeutic regimen can be called research on a human subject, without any stretch of the imagination, but this is *especially* so when little is known about the disease in question.

In my case there appears to be one indisputable fact: while the clinical picture is complex and confounding, every doctor I have spoken to, including Green, is one hundred per cent agreed on one point – the Arnold-Chiari malformation and its effects are barely, if at all, understood. Green's commitment to this diagnosis therefore carried an unusually heavy load of responsibility, because the presence of this anomaly would obliterate even further the gossamer line between the normal practice of medicine on the one hand and research on the other. Under these circumstances, any intervention which Dr. Green undertook, or failed to undertake, is ethical *only* if performed, or not performed, with my fully informed consent. To be considered informed a decision must be based on all the known, relevant information. When the doctor exercises his discretion, it must be consistent with whatsoever disclosure of fact is necessary to informed consent.

Let's face it, one of life's sternest lessons is that there is just no way you can eat your cake and have it too. Over and above all else, however, doctors have to do everything that is humanly possible to ensure that no intervention is undertaken or conducted *negligently*.

Another effect of imprudent litigation might be that doctors become reluctant to attend to patients in emergency situations, except upon the direct request of the patient, or where there is an existing professional relationship with the patient, or where there is a legal duty upon the doctor to act, as in the case of a doctor employed in the casualty department of a hospital, for example. One of the lesser consequences could be a rise in fees, brought about by the higher liability insurance premiums being passed on by the medical profession to the patient.

Ironically, then, it could be the general public – whose members may under certain circumstances legitimately endeavour to obtain redress against medical practitioners – who in the end are the real losers. Some might even go so far as to argue that it would be better for a few unfortunate malpractice victims to fall by the wayside, rather than to scare the whole medical profession into over-cautious inefficiency. In the United States, for example, the majority of state legislatures have already felt themselves constrained to introduce positive legislation in order to encourage doctors to act in emergencies. These enactments, known as Good Samaritan laws, make provision for the indemnity of licensed physicians who in good faith provide emergency medical treatment to unknown patients.

From very early times the doctor has been held responsible where want of care and skill has existed in the practise of medicine, since "it is the duty of every artificer to exercise his art rightly and truly as he ought".[1] The medical man's duty of care, then, arises quite independently of any contract with his patient. It is based simply upon the fact that the physician has undertaken the care and treatment of the patient. The sole guarantor of medical responsibility down the ages has been traditional ethics, which were originally enshrined in the Hippocratic Oath. However, the purely ethical foundation of medical law has been gradually supplemented by an increasingly rigid, complex and demanding judicial structure. The duty of care is a duty in the law of delict, and in the case of a doctor this exists even where there is a contract between him and the patient. An action against the physician is generally brought on the basis of delict, rather than for a breach of contract. Unless there is an express provision regarding the duty to be expected of the doctor, the implied contractual duty of care is virtually the same as the duty which exists in delict, namely a duty to exercise reasonable care in the circumstances.

The duties of a doctor and of medicine have become more closely defined. These legal offshoots of contemporary development are the counterpart of the transactions between modern medicine and a public rendered more demanding by the cost of medical care. In a modern society medicine has become a real public service, with all its consequent obligations. For some time past the doctor's life has been increasingly closely linked to a system of diverse and precise obligations that have only a superficial resemblance to the traditional ethical system. The medical ideal remains what it has always been, but more rigid legislation has developed, and will continue to do so. We are no longer in an age in which the doctor-patient relationship is based on the purely delictual duties of the doctor; we have arrived at the stage at which the patient believes – correctly, I

1. Nathan, H. L.: *Medical Negligence: Legal Case Studies.* London, Butterworth, 1957, p. 6.

think – that he has rights over medicine. If today's patient wants contraception she must be approached from the medical point of view and not that of the moralist. The doctor is obligated to enlighten her, regardless of his personal commitment, if the Pill is not to be subjected to commercial abuse. The priority, however, is that access to a system – and, as a corollary, to those who are voluntarily members of that system – that will help people *to achieve and maintain health* is a *right* of all citizens, and not a privilege of race, colour, creed, affluence or anything else.

The dignity of man has long been acclaimed in the arts, literature, painting and music. However, the courts have far to go in the recognition of the dignity of man – at least where personal injuries are involved. Man's political freedom was wrested from the rack, the thumbscrew, the wheel, solitary confinement. These and other forms of entrapment of the helpless or unpopular left their wake of crushed bodies and shattered minds along the way to the cross, the guillotine, the stake, the hangman's noose. And those who have suffered most have always been the poor, the ignorant, the numerically weak, the friendless and the powerless. Man has had the same struggle in gaining his economic freedom. The economic guarantees envisioned at the dawn of the industrial revolution were for years to come only mirages. Freedom from hurt and poverty and hunger did not simply flow from man's inventive genius as he conquered metal and steam and electricity. That freedom, too, had to be fought for. And the right of dignity of life and limb, breast and brain, has also to be fought for in the courts of law, and that fight is only just beginning.

Personal injury through medical malpractice can be a personal holocaust, a physical, mental and economic catastrophe. It can beggar the rich, and destroy the poor. Left in the wake of the doctor's negligence are those who will never again be free of pain, amputees, paraplegics, spinal injury invalids, the blinded and the burned – and those who suffer internal injuries, slow to manifest themselves and often difficult to diagnose, that set up chain reactions to destroy the victim's health. How much are *your* eyes worth? *Your* leg? *Your* heart? *Your* nervous system? *Your* mind? What price the psychological trauma, the mental anguish consequent upon hasty marriage, mischievous electro-shock therapy, wayward myelography? The time is now more than ripe to hammer out precise concepts regarding the rights that the patient has, as well as the nature and the form of the changing relationship between the doctor, the patient and the law.

It is, of course, the factor of good faith that lies at the core of every allegation of malpractice. A fundamental issue in my particular case is whether the doctor's refusal to answer the telephone, or his failure to return calls, even after a bitter harangue on the subject by the patient, and even when he knows that a disease as serious as multiple sclerosis is suspected by a colleague – a neurosurgeon comparably qualified, a man more mature, with longer experience, equally esteemed by other doctors, and, moreover, one against whom I have heard not a single derogatory report from a patient – is a bona fide error. Is the refusal to take into account this diagnosis of a crippling, incurable disease of the nervous system, the failure to refer the patient to a second colleague in the same city who is widely known to have a special interest in the disease in question, a bona fide mistake? I do not need recourse to a court of law or to an ethics committee, or to anyone, to find the answer to these and many similar questions that arise out of the conduct of the case. Neither is a bona fide mistake: both represent the most blatant and callous disregard of the fundamental rights of the patient. Both constitute a total breach of that tensile bond of trust that must be formed between the doctor and his patient if the latter is to be restored to health – for no patient should ever, in any circumstances, have the slightest doubt about her ability to rely utterly on the trust she places in her doctor, and most particularly where this trust has been expressly acknowledged. It is impossible to avoid the conclusion that both these actions also indicate moral turpitude, involving as they do a base neglect of the private and social duties man owes his fellow man.

Today the relationship between a patient and his doctor is essentially contractual, arising out of an express or implied agreement. Both parties must consent to the contract. The physician-patient relationship begins when the physician, in response to an express or implied request that he treat the patient, undertakes to render services; that is, a doctor-patient relationship does not exist unless the doctor contemplates treatment, thereby assuming responsibility for the medical care of the other person. After the relationship has been entered into, the physician is under an obligation to attend to the case as long as it is necessary to do so, unless he gives notice of his intention to withdraw from it, or is dismissed by the patient. One of

113

the prime elements of a negligence action is the existence of this legal duty of the physician to the injured party. While the contract relies on consent, and either party may terminate it at will, a physician cannot withdraw from a case and relieve himself of liability simply by staying away or abstaining from action, particularly if it turns out that, according to the standards of good medical practice, the patient requires further care. Where a duty of care once exists, liability attaches not only to a negligent act, but also to a negligent failure to act. If the physician does wish to withdraw from a case, he must give the patient reasonable notice of his intention to do so, and not abandon the patient until a replacement can be found. The physician may be held to have abandoned his patient by his lack of attention where this leads to an avoidable deterioration of the latter's condition. He can also be held responsible if he fails to see the patient as frequently as the requirements of good medical care dictate and where damages result from his failure.

In broad effect, the net result of the clash between the capitalistic urge and the crushing and compounding complexities of medical science on all fronts is that doctors are demanding, and getting, the best of two worlds: even if one keeps in mind the onus of the widespread socialisation of medicine, it is apparent that a ridiculously large number of patients pass through a doctor's hands each day, presumably filling the coffers to the desired level, and the doctor is by his badge of high office virtually protected from any liability for those acts of negligence that are inevitable under excessive duress. This state of affairs gives rise to a strong suspicion - fed by ample personal experience, as well as the stories that responsible men and women in every walk of life continually relate concerning the professional conduct of some doctors - that the largest oppressed minority today are the sick. Surely, then, the time has come to challenge the power of the medical profession? Surely it is clear that its members must be made insecure to *some* degree if they are to become more responsible?

3

The usual instruments of change in any organisation or social institution are external pressures: regulation, litigation, exposure to public opinion. But the adequacy and effectiveness of *any* of these is directly dependent on the internal freedom of those within the fraternity to act in accordance with the dictates of social conscience. This applies equally to the South African Medical and Dental Council, which is a regulatory body composed essentially of members of the fraternity whose conduct it was created to regulate. I know that its rulings on ethical and professional matters are law to the medical practitioner, and that doctors are inclined to view a charge before the Council in a more serious light than a criminal prosecution. Further, the creation of the body appears to be an attempt by the medical profession to set its house in order, and as a patient I am gratified by any effort on the part of the doctors to give me a better deal. But notwithstanding the existence of the Council, and regardless of whether the law is amended in some way – perhaps by invoking new legal tools in malpractice actions or by liberalising the concept of expert testimony – or whether malpractice cases are removed altogether from ordinary civil courts, the moral imperative must first be acknowledged by medical practitioners. More importantly, it must be acted upon. A greater freedom within the profession itself is essential to a creative insecurity amongst those who practise medicine, an insecurity that will generate a more suitable climate of responsiveness to patient interest and patient rights than that which prevails at present.

But if the doctors will not respond to the cry of the man in the street, if they remain impervious to the pressures of the humanistic decree and the twinge of social conscience, what then? The present situation in countries where Anglo-American rules governing court procedure and the giving of evidence apply is not satisfactory. Patients who have genuinely suffered damage as a result of medical negligence are entitled to fair compensation, but under current conditions they are largely prevented from seeking justice by the unwillingness of members of the medical profession to act on their behalf as expert witnesses. Once the precedence of the social good over professional camaraderie has been acknowledged, therefore, the first step could be to amend the law.

In the United States doctors are being sued in increasing numbers by their patients, and American case law on malpractice affords a rewarding field of study. According to Strauss there are few problems involving physicians that have not been the subject of a well-reasoned judgment in America, and courts elsewhere have not hesitated to follow these precedents. American case law emphasises the personal inviolability of the patient, and the courts are not inclined to place the physician on a pedestal. Thus in many states the defendant doctor has to share with other, non-medical, defendants the discomforts of *res ipsa loquitur* – the legal doctrine whereby harmful consequences in themselves may lead to an inference of negligence, unless the defendant can convince the court that he was not negligent. The damage or injury must be of such a nature that it would ordinarily not occur except for negligence. Then *res ipsa loquitur:* the occurrence itself is said to speak of negligence on the part of the defendant. This does not necessarily mean that the burden of proof has shifted to the defendant. However, should he fail to give a reasonable explanation for the events, the court might readily come to the conclusion that he was negligent. The duty of the defendant to explain is the cornerstone of the doctrine. In the United States "the courts have become more acutely aware of the need to protect an injured patient by inducing the physician to explain the reason for the injury and suffer the penalty of an adverse inference in the absence of such an explanation." [1] The doctrine has developed more or less into a rule of sympathy for patients in order to combat the conspiracy of silence among doctors.

The *res ipsa* principle covers the type of situation where the injurious result is manifestly in complete discord with the recognised therapeutic objective and technique of the operation or treatment involved. For example: cases where a swab, gauze or other material or instrument remains in a patient after surgery; where X-ray burns have been suffered during diagnosis; where infection has followed surgery or treatment; where burns have been inflicted by a warming bottle in an unconscious patient's bed; where a healthy organ (or tissue) adjacent to the diseased organ (or tissue) has been injured; and where an organ not in the area of operation has been injured.

Courts in both England and South Africa have almost consistently refused to allow a plaintiff in a malpractice case to rely on the

1. Strauss, S.A.: "The physician's liability for malpractice: a fair solution to the problem of proof?" *S.A. Law J.*, 419, 1967, p. 422.

doctrine of *res ipsa loquitur*. In 1924, in the leading case in South Africa of Van Wyk v. Lewis, the Appellate Division expressly refused to apply *res ipsa*. The defendant, a surgeon, had performed an urgent and difficult operation upon the plaintiff. At the conclusion of the operation one of the swabs used had been overlooked and remained in the plaintiff's body, from which it had passed after a lapse of twelve months. It was argued on behalf of the plaintiff that the fact that the swab was found in her body throws the onus on the defendant to prove that it was not left there negligently, or at least to explain the presence of the swab.

The question of onus is of capital importance. The general rule is that he who asserts must prove; a plaintiff who charges negligence must therefore establish it. If, at the conclusion of the case, the evidence is evenly balanced, he cannot claim a verdict, for he will not have discharged the onus resting upon him. However, in this case it was submitted that the mere fact that a swab was sewn up in the plaintiff's body is *prima facie* evidence of negligence, thereby shifting the onus onto the defendant to rebut the presumption. The *res ipsa* maxim was invoked in support of this contention.

On behalf of the defendant, however, it was argued that there had been no shift of onus. The plaintiff alleged a lack of reasonable care and skill, and the correctness or otherwise of that allegation could only be determined on a consideration of all the facts. There is no absolute test: it depends upon the circumstances. The nature of the occurrence is an important element, but it must be considered along with the other evidence in the case. It was held by the judge of appeal that it was impossible to appreciate the position, and to visualise, even imperfectly, the circumstances attending an abdominal operation of this nature without studying the mass of medical evidence placed before the court. Thus, in his opinion, the onus of establishing negligence rested throughout the case on the plaintiff. In short, if the surgeon is only liable for reasonable skill and care, and if the question of whether he acted reasonably or not depends upon all the accompanying circumstances, as far as the term reasonable is relative, the burden of proof must necessarily lie upon the plaintiff all the time. That is, the maxim *res ipsa loquitur* cannot apply where it depends upon something relative, not absolute, whether there was negligence or not. As soon as all the surrounding circumstances have to be taken into consideration, there is no room for the maxim. The plaintiff asserts negligence and bases his claim upon it, and this can only be determined by an examination of all the circumstances. Yet in other types of cases, specifically in road traffic sequels, courts have had few qualms about upholding this principle, thus demanding of the person who caused an injury to explain away his negligence.

In their substantial examination of South African medical law, published in 1967, Strauss and Strydom consider those circumstances that, in their view, justify the application of the principle of *res ipsa loquitur*. They hold that the unequivocal rejection of the maxim in the case of Van Wyk v. Lewis is not acceptable: such rejection clearly rests on an erroneous association of onus of proof and *res ipsa loquitur*. In a 1962 decision of the Appellate Division in Arthur v. Bezuidenhout and Mieny "the well-known distinction between an *onus* of proof and an obligation to adduce evidence"[1] was correctly emphasised. According to the judge in this case, *res ipsa loquitur* simply means that "proof by a plaintiff of an event properly falling within the maxim - that is to say, proof of an event which, in the absence of anything to the contrary, tells its own story - may justify an inference of negligence of the defendant. But that inference may be displaced by the remainder of the story: if the remainder of the story does not do so, then the inference remains - *res ipsa loquitur*. But the Court is not called upon to decide the issue of negligence until all the evidence is concluded, until it has heard all the story which there is to hear."[2]

It is difficult, I believe impossible, to counter the argument of Strauss and Strydom that leaving a swab inside a patient is so highly unusual and so utterly contrary to the therapeutic objective and technique of an operation that "it tells its own tale". Furthermore, the message it carries cannot be mistaken: it is one of negligence, gross and inexcusable negligence. What possible reasonable alternative explanation can there be for the presence of surgical miscellania inside the body of a patient after an operation? Is there any more eloquent example of the violation of the human body by an execrable want of care on the part of the medical practitioner and his assistants? The remark by the judge in Van Wyk v. Lewis that for the doctor to rebut a presumption of negligence is such a diffi-

1. Strauss, S.A. and Strydom, M. J.: *Die Suid-Afrikaanse Geneeskundige Reg.* Pretoria, J. L. van Schaik Bpk., 1967, p. 279.
2. *Ibid.*, p. 279.

cult task "in view of the lapse of time between operation and trial" does not convince the legal minds of Strauss and Strydom, and one can hardly expect that it will be understood by the layman: that is, by the individual most intimately involved, the victim or potential victim of an act of medical negligence. It is not merely difficult for the patient to explain what has happened during an operation: it is impossible. For one thing, the patient rarely has the requisite expert knowledge; but what is even more important, he is unconscious during surgery. Equity *demands* that the patient should merely have to establish a causal relationship between the doctor's act and the injurious consequence, and that it will then be for the doctor to provide a reasonable explanation of what occurred. In the absence of such an explanation, the patient ought to succeed with his action. What constitutes a reasonable explanation must be assessed *ex post facto* upon consideration of all factual circumstances. The doctor must show that he had applied every precaution that would reasonably be applied by the average practitioner of the same branch of medicine in order to avoid the untoward result.

Nonetheless, *res ipsa* does not provide a complete solution to the plaintiff's problems. Before the principle can come into operation, there must be proof of an injurious result caused by the defendant. In many cases, the injury and its cause may be so complicated that only an expert can explain the matter satisfactorily to the court. One of the principal difficulties in malpractice cases, of course, is the fact that they frequently involve controversial theories, and an expert witness might be called upon to make a choice which it would not be easy to justify. In order to establish a *prima facie* case and to avoid a verdict of "absolution of the instance", it might therefore still be necessary for the plaintiff to fortify his own story with expert medical evidence.

Although courts generally insist on expert evidence to prove negligence, some courts have decided against doctors in the absence of such evidence, simply on the grounds that it is "common knowledge" in society that a reasonable doctor would have acted differently. This doctrine, which has evolved in American law, is closely related to *res ipsa loquitur*. The rationale is simply that certain facts are so commonly known that a court may take cognizance of them and need not rely on expert witnesses to prove them. Obviously, it is applicable only in a limited number of extreme cases; one such instance is where a patient suffered temporary blindness as a result of an overdose of drugs administered by a nurse who had failed to follow the doctor's written instructions. However, it is an indication of a distinct trend towards ascribing absolute liability to medical practitioners. Many people do argue that the liability of the physician should be absolute, by analogy with the consumer movement, which is intent on uncovering the manufacturer's liability for defective products. And, indeed, the harder the doctor leans on the science, as opposed to the art, of medicine, the more his right to err diminishes. Some twenty-five years ago, if a patient died because his physician had administered Rh-incompatible blood, there was no negligence on the part of the physician. He had never heard of an Rh factor, never mind a test for determining its presence. Today, giving a blood transfusion without first testing the blood for this factor (that of both the donor and the receiver) would constitute gross malpractice. All this leads to a belief in a doctor's causal responsibility, apart from his ethical and intellectual responsibility; one step further, and we find the menacing presumption of collective causal responsibility. This formidable prospect, as well as some of the undeniable excesses in malpractice litigation in America, can only be avoided if, on the one hand, it is recognised that the single acceptable basis for professional liability is negligence, and if, on the other hand, the medical profession collaborates to the fullest extent in the search for more equitable protection for both patient and practitioner.

The plaintiff's difficulty in obtaining expert evidence has been solved in some degree in a few states in America by legislative amendments that enable the plaintiff to rely on recognised text books in providing a claim, without the necessity of calling an expert to agree with the passage on which reliance is placed. Nowadays there are excellent books on the market, explaining in simple language, tailored specifically to the lawyer's needs, the ramifications of traumatic medicine, for example, but these are not *per se* admissible as evidence in South Africa. Further, the crucial passage in a standard text may be so technical that its significance is lost without elucidation by an expert. There is also the strong possibility that the defendant himself or his expert witness may reject the treatise from which the statement is drawn as outdated or erroneous, and the plaintiff is rarely, if ever, in a position effectively to challenge such rejection.

Aid could also be given a plaintiff by being less strict about what is required for a medical practitioner to qualify as expert witness. Thus practitioners who are not within the same branch of medicine as the defendant could be permitted to testify in some cases. American courts have also allowed the plaintiff to go outside the immediate locality of the defendant's practice to obtain his experts, thus expanding the "same locality" standard to a "similar locality" standard. Nevertheless, these relaxations are of no avail where in a particular case no medical practitioner, whether in another branch of practice or in another locality, is available as witness.

4

Any forum other than the courtroom for dealing with an allegation of medical malpractice should, ideally, conform to five criteria. First, a patient injured while receiving medical care should receive adequate financial compensation. Secondly, the medical practitioner should be spared the emotional and financial stress of having to defend baseless suits. Thirdly, the claims for injuries should be processed quickly. Fourthly, costs should be controlled in such a way that neither defendant nor plaintiff pays excessive legal fees or other charges which are then passed on to the public. Lastly, there should be feedback from the operation of the system, whatever it is, to improve the quality of medical care. This appears to be the watershed between a viable alternative to current litigation and one which is not viable, from the point of view of each member of the triumvirate of doctor, lawyer and patient.

No matter what system is adopted, it must support the orderly development and publicising of legal criteria whereby a physician's conduct may be measured. The analysis of the medical practitioner's conduct in a given situation and the resulting publication of an opinion as to how this conforms to accepted standards of practice is the fundamental source of guidelines for other physicians who are involved in similar situations, and for their lawyers. It also constitutes the single comprehensive basis for delineating human rights in personal health care.

This is a vexed question, particularly in South Africa, on two counts. For one thing, our surgeons have pioneered human organ transplantation, and the future success of this enterprise is closely linked to commensurate legal enlightenment. Personal health care is the help in sickness that one man can give to another by virtue of his special skill and knowledge, or by donating blood or an organ. Such gifts to a fellow being can be considered the height of generosity. However, much more than benevolence is involved, since to declare something a right is to imply that the associated obligations can, and will, be met. The most serious difficulties of homo-transplantation arise in cases where this can occur only after the death of the donor.

The fundamental principle of medical ethics is to save life, and in this final quarter of the twentieth century an important life-saving resource is cadaver organs, in particular the liver and the heart, although only the latter generates emotive heat. The law too, of course, is deeply protective of human life. But paradoxically, now that medical science can prolong life with these organs, or at least alleviate suffering, the existing legal doctrine is not congruent with the fundamental policy of preserving life. The legal requirement that surgeons obtain the consent of the next of kin before removing organs from a cadaver is an obstacle to the routine transfer of organs from a lifeless body that has no use for them to live human beings who will die without them. Under these circumstances, cadaver organs that ought to be salvaged to aid the living become instead "flesh given to the worms". In short, if a sick man lacks access to either the skill and knowledge of the physician, or to any of the fund of life-preserving resources, he is being denied the possibility of being helped by means of some form of appropriate medical intervention.

The primary issues are *what* claims to cadaver organs, by *what* persons, should be recognised and protected by law. The decision must take into account several principles, the most important being the protection of the bodily integrity of a living person who still has a chance to live. Leaving aside the controversial question of when a person is alive and when he is dead, I think that cadaver organs should be used whenever they are needed to save the life of a living person. Where an individual or his kin forbid the use of cadaver organs, it must be asked whether either ought to have the right to deny life to another. Obviously, the salvaging of these organs must be done in such a way as to minimise the traumatic effect of the practice upon bereaved relatives, and under conditions that do not

122

burden the bereaved with the problem. In France, for instance, cadaver organs may be removed without the permission of the family, except from victims of crimes or accidents occurring at work, and from suicides and Moslems. Religion, or the customs of any racial or ethnic group, must be taken into account. Although in the distant past the Christian church shackled many advances in medical science, modern church doctrine is not opposed to cadaver transplants. In 1956 Pope Pius XII, in an address to an international meeting of ophthalmologists, declared that there could be no moral or religious objection to the post-mortem removal of the cornea for grafting purposes. The cadaver may be put to the use of the living so long as the body is treated with the respect due to "the one-time abode of a spiritual and immortal soul".

The Jewish position is more difficult to state authoritatively. On historical grounds many orthodox rabbis oppose autopsies, invoking a principle that the body must not be violated and that all parts of the body must be buried. However, it may be that the Jewish objections to autopsies do not apply to organ transplantation. Rabbi Simon Dolgin of the orthodox Beth Jacob congregation in Beverley Hills believes that organ transplantation from cadavers is permissible. His reasons are two-fold: saving a human life is paramount to all other laws; permitting cadaver transplants does not violate the rule that the deceased should be buried, since the organs will eventually come to rest, although in a different body. His views appear to be in agreement with those of most, though not all, rabbinical scholars.

The other difficulty in delineating human rights in health arises out of the fact that great cultural variations exist between the different patterns of medicine in the South African society. It has also to be borne in mind that this is a developing, and not a developed country.

In principle, civil (and political) rights anywhere can generally be secured by fairly simple legislation. Social and economic rights, on the other hand, require something more than this. The government has to have access to great capital wealth, and despite South Africa's undeniable affluence, it cannot yet command the resources that would guarantee each one of its inhabitants comprehensive social welfare. Which of the possible interventions in any system of medicine constitute a human right have therefore to be defined in terms of some set of criteria. For example: is one particular combination

123

of drugs, say, penicillin and streptomycin, "good medicine" for the newborn baby with septicaemia, under certain socio-economic circumstances, or would another combination, such as ampicillin and doxacillin, be better, due regard being given to the level of development of the system of health care at a particular point in time?

It is therefore pragmatic, though admittedly not wholly satisfactory, to proceed from intervention to rights, and not vice versa, because it is only in terms of intervention that human rights in personal health can be defined and handled. The starting point is the intervention that is needed for the person to achieve that state of health which is his by right. Clearly, therefore, we *must* retain the concept of negligence as the basis of professional responsibility if we are to make any kind of headway with the problem of defining the various rights and obligations of the patient and the medical practitioner.

Guidelines for judging the physician's conduct are clearly of the essence where a determination of fault, or want of care, is a condition of liability; preferably, *the* condition of liability. For example, from recent court decisions in two states in America has emerged the rule that physicians should seek consultation in cases that are difficult or beyond their competence. This rule comports with the Hippocratic Oath and is highly desirable. Its elevation to a virtual rule of law promotes the improvement of medical care and assists in the definition of substandard care. These guidelines play a quintessential role in formulating the most equitable relationship between the doctor, the patient and the law. They also emphasise the shortcomings of alternatives like arbitration and no-fault insurance as solutions to medical malpractice. Both of these were strongly recommended by a conference on malpractice held under the auspices of the United States Department of Health, Education and Welfare in 1971.

The first alternative, arbitration, allows parties to agree in advance to settle any disputes that may arise among them by participating in a relatively informal, non-judicial proceeding. An arbitration agreement may provide that, in the event of a claim, each party shall select an arbitrator and that the two arbitrators so chosen shall select a third. The panel of three then receives evidence relating to the claim and makes a decision. If the claim is found to have merit, the arbitrators determine the sum due to the plaintiff, or claimant. If not, the claimant receives nothing. The decision of the arbitrators is usually final and not subject to appeal to the courts, unless the parties agree in advance to allow appeals against adverse rulings.

There has been little experience with arbitration as a means of handling malpractice claims. In California two large medical groups and a few hospitals have adopted binding arbitration programs. Under these plans the general approach is to offer the patient an opportunity to sign an agreement stating that he is willing to submit possible future claims to arbitration, and to afford him a period of grace after signing in which he may rescind. When this period expires, the agreement becomes binding. The medical group that has the longest experience with arbitration apparently regards it as a successful alternative to conventional litigation. Nevertheless, it is difficult to accept that a patient who signs an arbitration agreement in the course of a hurried admission to hospital for treatment of a life-threatening illness, or because of injury through accident, is in any position to protect his legal right to bring suit for negligence or other forms of medical misdemeanour.

The second alternative is a no-fault professional liability program. This is, in effect, a means of deciding who should bear the expense of an unfortunate injury, and as such it entirely replaces the negligence standard for professional liability. It might, for example, provide that the patient carry his own insurance, and if he sustains an injury in the course of medical care, he would then file claim with his own insurer. If the claim is covered by the policy, he would be compensated for medical and hospital expenses and other out-of-pocket expenses related to the injury. He would generally retain the right to sue for extra damages in specific circumstances. These might include his having experienced an unusual amount of pain and suffering, or having incurred expenses not covered by the standard policy, or especially flagrant misconduct by a physician, such as amputating the wrong part.

Certainly this is not merely a rehash of all the old chestnuts in malpractice, which go back now a hundred years in the literature of medicine and law, but it may be seriously doubted whether either a system of arbitration or a no-fault system can deal effectively with the tortuous intricacies of the "malpractice crisis" that exists in the United States, and which I believe also exists in South Africa.

A compromise between amending the existing law, on the one hand, and removing malpractice actions from civil courts to have them adjudicated upon by special tribunals, on the other hand, could be found in medical malpractice screening panels. While the exact composition and function of these panels vary from place to place in the United States, the object is to make available, both to the patient who feels aggrieved, and to the physician whose treatment is disputed, a platform on which the problem may be brought nearer to a solution without the expense and publicity of a court proceeding. The opinions these panels issue are merely advisory, except in New Jersey. Nowhere is a patient compelled to submit his claim to the panel instead of proceeding to court.

A joint screening panel consists of both physicians and attorneys appointed by the medical society and bar association of the area. The number of members of the panel varies, as do other aspects of procedure, but the fundamental objective is the same wherever these panels exist. Either side may request that the panel hear the matter. If the plaintiff initiates proceedings, or agrees to the panel's acting, he must furnish all medical and hospital records without a claim of privilege - legal jargon for saying "we admit nothing and we establish no precedent". The hearing is usually quite informal and deals with whatever material each side wishes to present. Normally the panel members arrive at one of two decisions: that there is evidence that the physician was negligent and the patient was harmed by the negligence, or that there is no such evidence. Some panels have a third option. They may refuse to make a determination on the grounds that insufficient evidence has been presented to them. Where the panel finds in favour of the patient, it does not consider such matters as the quantum of damages that ought to be awarded.

If the decision of the panel is that there was no negligence involved in the treatment of the patient, it apparently serves to discourage legal action, even though the patient is not bound by this determination. If, on the other hand, the panel rules in favour of the patient, the medical society agrees to make an expert witness available to him if he proceeds with the matter. The indications are that most cases in which the panel finds negligence on the part of the physician are settled out of court. In those areas where joint screening panels are in use, both the medical society and bar association are apparently pleased with the result.

A screening experiment that is regarded as particularly successful was initiated in Manhattan in 1971. All medical liability suits are submitted to a panel of mediators consisting of a senior judge of the court, a personal injury lawyer and a physician specialising in the particular field of medical practice involved in the claim. All mediators serve without compensation. Each judge presiding over a panel is free to establish the procedure for the panel. In general, however, the case develops in three stages. First, complete medical and hospital records are furnished to the physician to study and analyse, the judge is given the complete file on the case, and the lawyer is given a copy of the pleadings and bill of particulars. Secondly, the panel meets for a hearing, for which one hour is allotted. The panelists meet by themselves for a preliminary discussion after the physician has explained the medical aspects of the claim. Lawyers for the parties then present the positions of their clients and are questioned, either together or separately, by the panelists. Thirdly, efforts are made to reach a mutually agreeable settlement between the parties. These activities vary greatly and may be conducted by the entire panel or by the judge alone. Final settlement often requires follow-up action, usually by the judge.

I have been given to understand that something along these lines has already been attempted in South Africa, and that the attempt failed. However, some such system is clearly preferable to extrajudicial tribunals or special courts. Strauss proposes that in every jurisdiction of this nature a medical investigator be appointed. His professional standing is seen as that of an experienced medical practitioner with a wide general knowledge of medical practice. As far as is necessary and expedient he would be assisted by full-time medical and legal experts, and an administrative staff. Alternatively, an advisory board could be constituted, and it would be the duty of every doctor to serve on such a board for at least twelve months during his professional career, much as members of the public were once liable for service on a jury. In either event, the primary task of the consultative agency would be to separate frivolous and vexatious claims against doctors from those based upon real and substantial grievances. An aggrieved person could lay his complaint before the agency in person or through a lawyer. However, a patient need not necessarily have recourse to such an agency; he would be quite entitled to institute an action directly in the civil courts.

The agency's proceedings would be informal and *in camera*. Any claim considered to be without merit would be rejected, with due regard to the information provided by the patient, and after such inquiries as might be deemed fit. This would, of course, not prevent the claimant from proceeding with an action against the doctor, should he so wish. Conversely, if the agency were satisfied that the claim was *prima facie* sound, it would pursue the investigation in all, or some, of several ways. First, the agency would appoint a panel of one or more medical experts (who would be under legal compulsion, in the same way as a witness in a civil case) to investigate the patient's complaint and examine him physically. Secondly, the complaint would be put to the defendant doctor, who would be invited to give an explanation, or make any statement he wished to make, or bring to the attention of the panel any fact he considered important. Thirdly, the panel would draw up a written report in which its findings would be set forth. Fourthly, the panel would be entitled at any stage of the proceedings to obtain such legal advice as it might require. Fifthly, in its report the panel would be entitled to comment on any medical or legal issue involved, provided that no comment is made on the quantum of damages. Finally, a copy of the report would be furnished to both the plaintiff and the defendant physician.

If the patient then decides to institute action, the panel's report would be handed in to the court. The defendant would, however, be entitled to challenge any allegation contained in the report as part of his case. He could do this either by cross-examining the investigator or by producing expert evidence to refute any statement in the report; he would not be entitled to cross-examine any of the medical experts who had served on the panel, although the presiding judge may permit this upon application by the defendant.

If this or some other parallel scheme is not acceptable, or cannot be implemented, the final resort would be to transfer malpractice litigation from the ordinary civil courts to special tribunals that have been empowered to adjudicate. These would be composed of both legal and medical experts who would examine the patient, the hospital records, the specialists' reports, the records of the defendant doctor - in short, an inquisitional process aimed at establishing the true facts. Like many other South Africans, I am bitterly opposed to the notion of "special courts", the first of which were introduced by the British during the Boer War, and it would indeed be unfortunate if in such a sensitive area steps in this direction were necessary. But as Professor Strauss so cogently points out, any citizen whose automobile has been tampered with in an attempted theft, or whose signature has been forged on a cheque, has at his disposal a well-equipped crime laboratory and an army of special investigators who will do their utmost to secure evidence that will bring the offender to justice. However, the citizen whose health has been impaired permanently or whose body has been injured irreparably because of a serious professional error on the part of his physician is nine times out of ten unable to lay his case before a court because of the unavailability of witnesses.

5

One critical question is raised by the difficulties that a charge of alleged medical negligence presents: what ways, if any, exist to exert the pressures necessary to induce the appropriate degree of concern among doctors for the rights of their patients? How do you rock the boat, if you believe in the name of humanity that it ought to be rocked?

The obvious course is concerted action by those who are ill. It is just as obvious why this is easier said than done. The ill are too old, too young, too inarticulate, too disabled, too dispirited, too vulnerable, too transient in existence, to constitute an effective lobby. They cannot parade, or chant slogans, or carry banners, or present briefs where they might do some good. They are too afraid to protest, because in *fact,* if not in law, the relationship between the doctor and the patient is *not* based on mutual consent: it is coercive, and it is coercive because his condition renders the patient dependent on his doctor. A relationship of consent between two persons where one is inherently dependent on the other, for whatever reason, is a contradiction in terms.

There is therefore no quieter, no more submissive, no more intimidated coterie than the sick. But when you consider the overwhelming power, sophistication and affluence, the polished organisation of the group that they are faced with, is it any wonder that there is scarcely a squeak from the sick? How, in this society, or in any other where the law is inimical to the welfare of this minority, can the wronged patient join battle with his physician? Apart from excursions of the pen, the answer is that he is virtually precluded from doing so. The doctor knows this, the lawyer knows it, and the victim of medical negligence knows it. The only way open is for the patient to lay his case directly before the public.

In my case the issues are fairly clear-cut, although the answers are obscure. Moreover, whereas a lawyer presents a case in order to win, the scientist cannot do so. Each pursues truth in his own accredited fashion.

In brief, the first issue is that of misdiagnosis. While a wrong diagnosis in itself can hardly render the doctor legally liable, according to Strauss and Strydom, it may be causally responsible for the use of inappropriate procedures, or for wrong treatment. Bearing in mind the fact that the symptoms of different diseases are sometimes almost identical, and that medical science may continuously "discover" new diseases and reactions, a wrong diagnosis may be made even where a thorough examination has taken place. Where a wrong diagnosis has been made, the doctor can be considered really blameworthy only if he did not examine the patient properly, or did not avail himself of the most efficient examination techniques, or undertook a diagnostic examination without sufficient knowledge.

In the South African case of Mitchell v. Dixon the Appellate Division in 1914 held that "a medical practitioner is not necessarily liable for wrong diagnosis. No human being is infallible: and in the present state of science, even the most eminent specialist may be at fault in detecting the true nature of a diseased condition. A practitioner can only be held liable in this respect, if his diagnosis is so palpably wrong as to prove negligence, that is to say, if his mistake is of such a nature as to imply an absence of reasonable skill and care in the profession."

In the 1958 English case of Crivon v. Barnett Group Hospital Management Committee and Others the patient's disease was wrongly diagnosed as cancer of the breast. The court held that there was a great difference of opinion on the interpretation of the microscope slides on which the diagnosis was based. The court asked whether, under the circumstances, it could be said "to be negligence in a pathologist, when he came to a conclusion which a great expert might himself have come to? When there was such a debatable field and such difficulty in interpreting these slides, it could not be said to be negligence for a pathologist to appear to have come to the wrong decision. The patient said he ought at least to have taken a second opinion since this was such a serious matter for her. Some people might say it would have been better: but once such a thing as this was diagnosed everyone knew that speed of treatment was essential. The mere fact that a second opinion was not taken and that there was no further additional check, for instance at the hospital, did not make out a case of negligence. Unfortunate as it was that there was a wrong diagnosis, it was one of those misadventures, one of those chances, that life held for people."

To paraphrase Hobbes, life is raw in tooth and claw, and we are fortunate if we complete the journey from the cradle to the grave unscathed. But surely science has progressed to the point where medical misadventures can be kept to a minimum?

However, for the plaintiff to succeed in a claim that he is the victim of something more than outrageous chance, it must be demonstrated that the diagnostic error which was coupled with the bad result was the product of substandard medical practice. Further, a direct causal relationship between the doctor's conduct and the injury that the patient sustains must be established. Proof must also be provided that a more perceptive diagnosis would probably have averted the bad result.

Multiple sclerosis is a disease in which symptoms and pathological lesions are disseminated in time, and in space, anatomically. Keeping in mind the complete history of my case at that time, was there enough evidence in December 1974 to suggest that I suffered from the disease? One doctor claims that there can be no doubt that there was: in his words, it is a florid case of multiple sclerosis. However, it is my opinion that Green did not think so. In the light of subsequent events it is pertinent to ask: if not, why not? Because of the myriad signs and symptoms? The implication, again keeping in mind the circumstances of the case at that time, is that the Arnold-Chiari malformation does present with such myriad signs and symptoms. On the other hand, Green may have harboured some suspicion of multiple sclerosis, and his line could have been that multiple sclerosis is an exclusion disease, and that this was why the myelogram was performed: in order to make quite sure that he was dealing with multiple sclerosis and not a surgically remediable lesion masquerading as a degenerative process. According to him, the X-rays confirmed his diagnosis of an Arnold-Chiari lesion. This decision was tentatively confirmed by a neurosurgeon in Johannesburg who is regarded as an expert on this congenital anomaly. But it is not supported by the radiologist's report, and no other neurologist, neurosurgeon or radiologist who has seen the plates has accepted that they support such a diagnosis.

The question of why the myelogram was done at all is interesting. It is said that ill-considered myelography often discloses more information about the examiner than it does about the patient. What, for example, did Green expect to learn about my defective vision by using this technique? Why was a less traumatic procedure not adopted in the first instance, such as referral to another neurologist?

Furthermore, I would not have given my consent for the myelogram had I been adequately appraised of the serious risk involved. Valid consent requires knowledge and appreciation of risks involved. While I accept that Green was probably motivated by my best therapeutic interest, his disclosure to me amounted to a statement that a myelogram is not painful, but that the removal of the dye is; this is not sufficient to assure informed consent, and it is not at all clear that another competent neurologist would have undertaken the same procedure in an analogous situation. Two neurologists have denied flatly that they would have done so.

When a physician conducts a diagnostic study or gives treatment that may injure the patient, he must obtain in advance the patient's informed consent. Failure to do so may give rise to a charge of professional liability, which may be based on negligence or on assault. It is difficult to determine what constitutes informed consent. In the United States the trend seems to be toward allowing the adequacy of the physicians's disclosure to be determined by laymen. The testimony of other physicians as to how much information they give their patients about a diagnostic test is not necessary where evidence exists concerning the nature and risks of the procedure. A doctor's failure to disclose, on the grounds that it was "for the good of the patient", whatever that may mean, is an infringement of the right of the patient to decide about what is done to his body. "Anglo-American law starts with the premise of thoroughgoing self-determination. It follows that each man is considered to be master of his own body, and he may, if he be of sound mind, expressly prohibit the performance of life-saving surgery, or other medical treatment. A doctor might well believe that an operation or form of treatment is desirable or necessary but the law does not permit him to substitute his own judgment for that of the patient by any form of artifice or deception."[1] The doctor who proceeds under the doc-

1. Justice Schroeder. Natan v. Kline. Quoted in Katz, J.: *Experimentation with Human Beings.* New York, Russell Sage, 1973, p. 85.

tor-knows-best theory, without securing a deliberate waiver from his patient and without disclosing collateral hazards, substitutes his judgment about the need for undergoing risk for that of his patient. This substitution is inconsistent with the respect the law has for the patient's control over his own body.

In any event, in a study of informed consent Alfidi found that patients will not refuse *indicated* but risky diagnostic procedures even where disclosure includes a description of the severest possible complications. The argument that fully informing a patient compromises his care can only be viewed with the greatest scepticism.

Green made no attempt whatsoever to elicit informed consent from me for either of the diagnostic procedures he undertook. I was extremely dubious about the necessity for the angiogram, and I would certainly have thought more carefully about it had I known that a stroke was a definite risk of the procedure. When I inquired specifically about the possible ill-effects I was told by Green, who illustrated his words by indicating a point midway on the left side of his neck with his index finger, that I might have "a bit of stiffness here, nothing more". As it turned out, he was right. In fact, the apparent lack of any effect at all, either from the myelogram or the angiogram, caused him to remark that I have a constitution like a horse.

Unfortunately, in the long run the outcome of the myelogram was not benign. This procedure involves a special danger of which I had no knowledge and of which I should have been made aware. I can state, without equivocation, that as the myelogram did not seem to be clearly indicated, I would under no circumstances have consented to the procedure *in the first instance* had I known of the risk to health which was involved, no matter how slight the degree of that risk. My experience with shock treatment has made me far too chary for that. I would have insisted upon a second opinion.

Thus, whether or not the myelogram and the angiogram were carried out with the utmost skill, as both were performed on a non-consenting patient, Green is liable on the basis of *iniuria*.

Myelography is a valuable and often essential aid in the diagnosis of intraspinal lesions, but the radio-opaque iodised compounds that are widely used for this purpose are not completely harmless, as is generally believed. The irritating effects of the injected compounds are caused by the tiny dispersed particles produced when the substance becomes emulsified, and it has been found that

Myodil becomes fixed in position in the subarachnoid space from within a few months to a year. Although the distribution within the cranial cavity varies, the globules of Myodil are most commonly seen in the basal cistern, in the floor of the anterior and middle fossae, and scattered throughout the posterior fossa. While there is no extensive clinical and experimental data that suggests that iodised oils contribute to severe and disabling arachnoiditis, sometimes resulting in death, there can be no reasonable doubt that in susceptible patients iodised oils are not without danger, and every precaution must be taken in their use. This includes sensitivity tests to determine possible allergy, and the removal of the contrast medium as soon as possible after myelography.

In my case, the Myodil was removed 211 days after its introduction into the spine. How much Myodil remained can be gauged from the X-rays taken by Dr. Peters. Both he and Green observed that there was "a lot" (although Rice did not agree), but I do not know whether this means an unusually large amount considering the length of its stay in the spine. The absorption of Pantopaque, which is a similar iodised oil used for the same purpose, is most rapid in the first few months after injection; the average rate of absorption is 0,5 ml in eleven months. The Myodil that remained in the spine may therefore be considered a foreign body, much as a swab sewn up in a patient is a foreign body. Its presence resulted in arachnoiditis, which was not treated – it was not even recognised – and cannot be treated now, and which has caused and still causes intractable pain and suffering.

At approximately 6.15 p.m. on Tuesday, 28th January, 1975, I heard your voice in the corridor outside my ward, Dr. Green, tell the sister, so neat in her trim blue uniform, so demure with her straight brown upswept hair, that you would have to get that dye *out*. I did not think you meant 211 days later. I am sure that neither did the sister, because she repeated your words verbatim when I reported that the spasms in the leg had continued unabated throughout the night. Why did you take so long, Dr. Green? What else did I have to do to drive home my point, to convince your sceptical mind that I was in agony, that I needed help, *your* help? Perhaps I would have been able to command the requisite care if I had lost the use of *both* my legs – although, somehow, I doubt it. That could only have meant that I was twice as neurotic. If the presence in my spine of an oil with a ravaging potential was no more than an unfortunate

oversight, a mere incident in the neurological scheme of things, re-
grettable but certainly not negligent, *where,* members of the sacred
brotherhood, *where,* ladies and gentlemen of the public, *where* in
the name of justice does the onus lie for proving this contention? If
the days and weeks and months to come are to be marred, as those
of the recent past have been, with prolonged and exquisite pain, if
that is the price that I have to pay for a medical misfeasance, surely
it is not too much to expect that Dr. Green should face the medical
man's nightmare, which may be the ultimate deterrent to the fickle
and feckless way the mandated task of care is fulfilled in consulting
rooms across South Africa: that is, the application in a court of law
of the legal maxim of *res ipsa loquitur* in the case of an allegation of
medical negligence. Will you please explain, Dr. Green, why the
assault on, why the rape of my nervous system was perpetrated in
the first place, and why it was then permitted to continue for seven
months, so that when it was all over, it was too late, and I was faced
with the prospect of permanent disability? And if Dr. Green is
unable to provide an adequate explanation, how, honourable members of the Bench, can I?

6

I am willing to grant that Green does exercise a measure of caution
in his use of diagnostic procedures. I accept, without qualification,
that he was sincere in his conviction that the angiogram was clearly
indicated by the circumstances of the case; and his sincerity, within
the context of what occurred in his surgery that day, overcame my
reservations concerning the appropriateness of that particular
procedure. However, about his decision to perform the myelogram
I concur with the spontaneous view expressed by Jill when she
heard of it: I believe that, bearing in mind his approach to the case
from the outset, her comment that "he is just trying to prove his
point" is fully justified. Green's obduracy about his initial impetuous
diagnosis of an Arnold-Chiari malformation appears to have dis-
torted his medical judgment, and I think that he threw professional
caution to the winds. I do not accept that the myelogram was
indicated beyond reasonable doubt and that consultation with

135

professional colleagues was therefore precluded, nor do I accept that it was performed with due regard to the risks involved.

Furthermore, while Green may observe some of the proprieties attached to diagnostic procedures, his approach to drug therapy is frankly cavalier. For one thing, he clearly does not recognise any need to monitor for toxicity. To minimise the chances of liability on their part, drug manufacturers generally take great care to inform physicians about the indications for and the risks attached to the use of their products. One way of doing this is by distributing well-illustrated, carefully detailed and clearly worded brochures. In a recent case in Minnesota it was alleged that a physician was negligent in the way he prescribed a particular drug and monitored for toxic side effects. The package insert for the drug was introduced into evidence, and other evidence indicated that the dose the physician prescribed and his following of blood counts varied from the recommendations of the package insert. In response to a brief filed by the state medical association, the state supreme court formulated a rule that a physician's deviation from the package insert is *prima facie* evidence of negligence if there is competent medical testimony that his patient's injury or death resulted from the doctor's failure to adhere to the recommendations.

The United States leads the world in the control of and legislation for the manufacture of drugs. The Food and Drug Administration requires that a pharmaceutical company prove not only the safety but also the effectiveness of a drug. That is, that the drug will not prove poisonous if used in the recommended doses, and that in addition it will be proved to the satisfaction of the authorities that it is effective. The view of this organisation is that "although labeling along with medical articles, tests and expert opinion, may constitute evidence of the proper practice of medicine, it alone is not controlling on this issue. The labeling is not intended either to preclude the physician from using his best judgment in the interest of the patient, or to impose liability if he does not follow the package insert. A physician should recognise, however, that the package insert represents a summary of the important information of the conditions under which the drug has been shown to be safe and effective by adequate scientific data submitted to the Food and Drug Administration."[1] In other words, the physician may use his best judg-

1. *FDA Drug Bulletin,* October, 1972.

ment, but he must be aware that the package insert or similar data may be used to attack his judgment.

Of the various drugs the neurologist prescribes, anti-convulsants seem to be those most likely to generate medicolegal problems. However, even if a drug is potentially lethal, or at the least deleterious, the act of prescribing it does not by itself create liability. There must be evidence that the specialist was negligent in his selection of it, that he failed to disclose side effects or toxicity and failed to observe for them, or that he was negligent in the way he managed an adverse reaction when this did occur. The doctor who prescribes an anti-convulsant may in various ways lay himself open to a charge of liability: by failing to inquire about previous adverse reactions, by prescribing without indication or in the face of a contra-indication, by failing to warn about symptoms of toxicity, by failing to monitor blood counts, and by failing to discontinue the drug despite an adverse reaction to it. A common side effect may initiate an unfortunate chain of events. There was the case of Kaiser v. Suburban Transportation System in Washington in 1965, where a physician had prescribed an antihistamine drug to a bus driver for a cold. The driver fell asleep at the wheel and ran into the plaintiff's car. The plaintiff recovered a judgment from the physician based on the latter's failure to warn the driver about the soporific effects of the drug.

The relevance of this case to the prescription of anti-convulsants, which often have a sedative effect, is pointed. I was one patient who experienced marked drowsiness not only at the commencement but throughout the course of anti-convulsant therapy. During the period when I was swallowing 1 200 mg of Tegretol per day, I drove my car only when circumstances forced me to do so. Dr. Rice never failed to press me to try to cut down the dosage. I tried repeatedly to do so, but I was unable to reduce the dosage by so much as one Tegretol (200 mg) per day due to the relief they afforded from the lower back and limb pain. However, as the toxic symptoms mounted, Dr. Evans finally forced me to discontinue the drug altogether, though nothing, apart from Pethidine, is as effective in combatting the attacks of pain. The function of Tegretol as an anti-convulsant in my case raises an interesting point. I have not taken an anti-convulsant of any kind since 29th December, 1975. However, control is obviously being exerted by means of other drugs which Dr. Evans holds to be effective in retarding the progress of multiple

137

sclerosis, and in ameliorating the effects of extant damage. Since beginning his treatment I have not fainted, nor have I had a fit, and there have been no indications that these phenomena will recur. Evans himself does not discount this possibility, but says it would surprise him very much.

The efficacy of Tegretol as an anti-convulsant seems to be established, but its depressant effects on the functioning of bone marrow and the formation of white blood cells require that it be used with care, which means obtaining the informed consent of the patient to its use in treatment, as well as constant supervision of the dosage. The latter is particularly important, since Tegretol may induce vertigo, along with other secondary effects. In a study of forty patients with trigeminal neuralgia, Dr. Blom of Uppsala, Sweden, received reports of this disturbance from twelve participants. In four of the cases the vertigo was experienced as severe. All four patients had multiple sclerosis. Apparently, trigeminal neuralgia – and temporal lobe epilepsy, where this exists – are sometimes symptomatic of multiple sclerosis. Like Dr. Green, I am a firm believer in clinical medicine.

7

Green's subsidiary diagnosis in my case was hysteria. The serious study of this disease began when Jean Charcot in 1862 became physician to the hospital of the Salpêtrière, where he founded the greatest neurological clinic of modern times. He was particularly interested in the hysterical patients at the clinic. Originally, hysteria had been supposed to be predominantly a female sexual disease: the Greek *hystera* means uterus. Charcot more or less adhered to the demonological belief that the possessed are more often female than male. At any rate, he once exclaimed in Freud's hearing that "in this kind of case it is always something genital – always, always, always".

Pierre Janet was Charcot's pupil and successor. As director of the psychological laboratory at the Salpêtrière, he systematised the body of clinical facts about hysteria and also brought them into line with some of the more generally understood concepts of psychology. From 1889 Janet emphasised the emotional causation of hysteria, relegating the sexual factor to the status of symptom rather than cause. He never quite got over his view of hysteria as a degenerative psychic phenomenon, and he still designated the major symptoms "stigmata". These were the anaesthesias, amnesias, abulias and motor disturbances, to which Janet added the accidents, the symptoms which occur irregularly – subconscious acts, fixed ideas, attacks, somnambulisms and deliriums. These develop by a psychic mechanism analogous to that of suggestion. Janet's main argument about hysteria was that it was a splitting of personality, caused by a concentration of the field of consciousness on one system of ideas and its retraction from others.

Sigmund Freud, who was also a pupil of Charcot, took his doctor's degree in 1881 and the following year began the private practice of neurological therapy in association with Joseph Breuer. When Freud joined him, Breuer had already tried treating hysterical cases with hypnosis and had discovered what he and Freud came to call catharsis, the "talking cure". One patient, a young girl with a great many symptoms, found her difficulties relieved after she had been induced under hypnosis to describe the emotional event which had brought on her trouble, and after she had given full expression to her feelings about it. Freud interpreted the mechanism of hysteria as the result of a psychic traumatism or nervous shock – fright, anxiety, shame, physical pain – of sexual nature initially, leading to morbid brooding and a kind of mental involution.

This psychical trauma, or rather the memory of the trauma, acts like a foreign body which, long after its entry, must continue to be regarded as an agent that is still at work. It operates in some way or other for years – not indirectly, through a chain of intermediate causal links, but as a directly releasing cause. "Hysterics suffer mainly from reminiscences."[1] However, these memories, unlike the other memories of their past lives, are not at the patients' disposal. On the contrary, they are completely absent when the patient is in a normal psychical state, and it is only on questioning under hypnosis that these memories emerge. In fact, when in a normal state psychically hysterics are generally people of the clearest intellect, strongest will, greatest character and highest critical power. Otherwise, however, they are insane. The difficulty with this is that the word "insane" is

1. Breuer, J. and Freud, S.: *Studies on Hysteria.* New York, Basic Books, 1957, p. 7.

not a term from either medical or scientific language; it is a popular term, or more accurately, the language of the law, although even here there is an increasing tendency to avoid its use. An insane person is an individual who is dangerous to others, or to himself, without being legally responsible for the danger he creates. This definition does not apply to the intrinsic characteristics of the disease, but to an extrinsic and accidental characteristic that depends on the situation in which the patient finds himself. The danger created by a patient depends much more on the social circumstances in which he is placed than on the nature of his psychological disorder. Such a distinction between insane and sane may be necessary for the safety of the public, but it does nothing to illuminate the disease.

There are two reasons why these traumatic memories do not fade and become forgotten. They may be attached to traumas which prevent a reaction in the patient, such as the apparently irreparable loss of a loved person, or where social circumstances make a reaction impossible, or they may concern matters which the patient wished to forget and therefore intentionally repressed from his conscious thought and inhibited and suppressed. Secondly, the traumas may have originated during the prevalence of severely paralysing affects, such as fright, or during positively abnormal psychic states, such as the semi-hypnotic twilight states of day-dreaming. The nature of these states makes reaction to the event impossible.

Unlike Charcot, who regarded the hypnotic state as a neurotic condition identical with hysteria, Breuer and Freud consider that the *sine qua non* of hysteria is the existence of hypnoid states: they provide the soil in which the affect plants the pathogenic memory with its consequent somatic phenomena. They often grow out of the day-dreams which are so common even in healthy people, "and to which needlework and similar occupations render women especially prone".[2] It is unclear why the pathologic associations formed in these states are so stable and why they have so much more influence on somatic processes than ideas are usually found to have; nevertheless, in terms of the Breuer-Freud formulation the products of hypnoid states intrude into waking life in the guise of hysterical symptoms.

The various hysterical symptoms, or ostensibly spontaneous

2. Breuer, J. and Freud, S.: *Studies on Hysteria.* New York, Basic Books, 1957, p. 13.

idiopathic products of hysteria, include neuralgias and anaesthesias, contractures and paralyses, hysterical attacks and epileptoid convulsions, chronic vomiting and anorexia, and constantly recurrent visual hallucinations.

The connection between the precipitating factor and the symptom may be quite evident in some circumstances; in others, it consists only in what is called a "symbolic" relation between the cause and the pathologic phenomenon – in the words of Breuer and Freud, a relation such as healthy people form in dreams. For instance, vomiting may follow on a feeling of disgust. However, in the case of the typical hysterical symptoms, such as hemi-anaesthesia, it is difficult to understand at first sight how they can be determined in this manner.

There can be little doubt that Sigmund Freud is the thinker who has made the greatest contribution to modern psychology; the only other possible contender is the Swiss Jean Piaget. However, Freud's school has occasioned abuses in medical practice, and he himself has lapsed into extravagances of rationalisation that can be described as giving rich reasons for poor motives. In psychoanalysis, Freud has invented an instrument that can be exceedingly dangerous in untrained – and a doctor who has not himself undergone analysis is untrained – and intemperate hands. I wonder how many women, every day, in how many surgeries, sit across from a doctor who has privately labelled them as hysterical. It is particularly unfortunate, from my point of view at any rate, that the organic nervous disease most likely to be confused with hysteria is multiple sclerosis, on account of the transitory occurrence in the early stages of this disorder of weakness and sensory disturbance. Moreover, certain organic diseases, especially multiple sclerosis, seem to predispose to hysteria. Then, too, typically hysterical symptoms may occur in patients with a focal abnormality of the temporal lobe, which according to the EEG readings exists in my case. It seems unnecessary to point out that calling them "typically hysterical symptoms" does not mean that they *are* hysterical symptoms. As one example: I have not been able to trace a single reference to Horner's syndrome appearing as a hysterical symptom, and it was Green himself who diagnosed my constricted right pupil as Horner's syndrome. Why, then, were further steps not taken to rule out the possibility of multiple sclerosis – particularly in view of the equivocal nature of the Chiari, to which Green admitted – by calling for further medical opinions, on *both* multiple sclerosis and hysteria? Why was a psychiatrist not called in? For even if Green is an authority in each area, he is certainly no expert on, or even superficially acquainted with, my psychic development or present state of mind.

However, it is an exercise in futility to attempt to evaluate the case. Before there can be any question of calling upon the defence to give evidence in answer to the plaintiff's claim, it must be reasonably certain that, on the plaintiff's evidence, there is a case for the defendant to answer. The whole burden of my argument, and my reason for setting it down in this way, is that it is precisely because of the extreme difficulty this decision presents to laymen - no matter how highly skilled in their respective specialities they are - that this case is not now before a court of law.

The question that my case raises, and that remains to be answered, is the question of liability for professional negligence: is this case of mistaken identity a case of negligent diagnosis, of such a nature as to imply an absence of reasonable skill and care on the part of Dr. Green, with due regard to the ordinary level of skill in the profession? In respect of his acts or omissions, did Green fail in his duty to the patient? Put another way: on the balance of probabilities, was there a breach of duty on the part of the defendant? Are the facts more consistent with an explanation of negligence than with any other explanation?

If the answer to this is yes, what steps will we take to ensure that another patient, in a similar position, will in future be able to seek and obtain redress for injury suffered as the result of medical malpractice?

Part III   A Pill for the Patient?

At a stage where much has been said, and a little has been done, to define and establish the rights of the patient, to protect the interests of the medical practitioner, we may well ask: will all be well for the patient once doctor, patient and law are marching more or less in step? Perhaps, if preventive medicine on a grand scale were a concrete reality, the answer could be yes. Unfortunately, the hard fact is somewhat different: a dominant concern with curative medicine and the wholesale specialisation of the profession can be foreseen in the immediate future. Specialisation in itself is not necessarily bad; the danger lies in its pronounced bias toward narrow technical skill, with a consequent decrease in generalist activities.

The technological approach in medicine is the application of scientifically grounded knowledge and techniques in a rational approach to the treatment of pathological states. The demand that this knowledge should be applied and distributed as medical services to as many people as possible means that, willy-nilly, medicine must shift from a relatively simple to a highly complex state where more and more people are required to perform more, and more differentiated, medical tasks. The point is whether this differentiation, coupled with the growth of the modern medical care system, does save more lives, does lengthen life expectancy, does reduce disability and suffering, does eliminate ever more pathological conditions, and so on.

Contrary to what one might expect, our health, in terms of sickness rates, has actually deteriorated in the past twenty years. In this period days off work for certified illness per one hundred men in Great Britain rose by 127%. Neither can we consider ourselves healthier if we take the costs and quantities of drug consumption as a barometer. In the United Kingdom there was a 25% growth in the number of prescriptions issued during the ten years 1959-1969. The clamour for psychotropic (or mood-altering) drugs, which tranquillise or sedate or elevate, and the tons of antibiotics prescribed are also indicative of a decline in public health. It is not impossible that this down-swing is to a great extent the result of adverse drug reactions. In 1973 the American Senate Sub-committee on Health heard evidence that according to the most conservative estimate of the Food and Drug Administration there are about one hundred Americans dying *every day* because of adverse drug reactions. Add to this an estimated three billion dollars per year for institutional care for those suffering these reactions, and an unexpected perspective on pill-popping emerges.

The mind boggles at the extent of our reliance on drugs. The financial strength of the drug companies, particularly of the giant international corporations, bears startling testimony to our medicinal gluttony. For many years now in the States the profits of the pharmaceutical industry have been twice the average for all other American industries, including the automobile industry. Make no mistake about it, there *is* gold in them thar pills. Of course, the goals of the drug industry, like those of every other profit-maximising enterprise, are commercial and not altruistic. But the industry is unique in that it has a market strength that is not, and cannot be, achieved by any other concern. Cosmetics and cars and clothes compete for the dollar, pound and rand on the basis of desirability, price and quality. The drug industry is not subject to this competitive struggle against other industries. I think few would dispute that the prescription has precedence over all other purchases.

Could it be, then, that it is the much vaunted pharmacological revolution - providing as it does for the treatment of diseases at various levels, from the underlying cause to its purely symptomatic manifestations - that has emasculated the doctor, rendering him less and less capable of *caring* for the sick? Does the fact that he has to see too many patients and is always in a hurry impel him to prescribe more and more industrially inspired drugs, thereby creating more and more disastrous effects and a burgeoning drug dependency, and finally driving more and more people, lemming-like, back to the doctor? For what? Another prescription, what else?

Today, the doctor is prescribing ever more to achieve ever less. Never before have so many swallowed so much to so little effect. For the sobering facts of life and death are unchanged: there has been no significant improvement in the treatment of that formidable array of killing diseases that wipe us out after the age of forty-five - the heart, lung and blood vessel diseases, and cancer.

Diseases like multiple sclerosis barely enter the picture at all. No cinderella complaint has the remotest hope of affecting the over-concentration of research by the cash-crazed drug industry into such profitable areas as mood-altering drugs. Remember: Thalidomide was prescribed as a sleeping pill or as a tranquilliser, and there can be no more horrific saga in the annals of medicine.

Everyone knows about Thalidomide babies, but few realise that the drug caused an estimated forty thousand[1] cases of polyneuritis in adults before it was withdrawn by its manufacturers. Polyneuritis is closely related to multiple sclerosis; both are incurable, degenerative diseases of the nervous system. Think about it - a tranquilliser has been proved capable of irreparably damaging the nerve fibres. If you cannot grasp the full import of this, and if you have never seen a Thalidomide baby, just walk into a room full of people who have multiple sclerosis. And give a moment's thought to these statistics, based on drug consumption in the United Kingdom *alone:* five years ago prescriptions for barbiturates reached twenty million per year; for phenylthiaxine tranquillisers, six million; for amphetamines, five million; for non-barbiturate hypnotics, five million. But who knows, the message here may be the medium: perhaps the doctor *is* making a valiant bid to salvage the rapidly eroding doctor-patient relationship with his prescription pad.

Whether we have reached the stage where the inordinate increase in our consumption of drugs is actively preventing genuine improvement in public health is difficult to assess. A major problem in the domination of the medical profession by the drug industry, and by technology generally, is certainly the doctor's neglect of the pathology for which no prescription can be given. More frightening, though, is the horrible truth that medicine - even if the production of psychotropic drugs were to quadruple - can no longer satisfy basic human needs. Doctors who believe - and they are legion - that what the patient *really* wants is the best technical medical care available, and that he will be satisfied with that, are perilously out of touch. Patients also want sympathetic care, and I think that most of them regard this as the most important aspect of the doctor's task.

Thus, while specialisation is unquestionably responsible for medicine's technical success, such as it is (after all, we are still stuck with

1. Sjoström, H. and Nilsson, R.: *Thalidomide and the Power of the Drug Companies,* London, Penguin Books, 1972, p. 92.

the common cold, never mind multiple sclerosis), it is also specialisation that is at the root of its tragic failures in the area of compassionate care. The suffering, frightened patient, and very often those near him, is vitally dependent on comfort, and on continued reassurance and support during the course of illness or disability, whether this is incurable or not. And this is not because he is mentally unhinged either, Dr. Green and dozens of other specialists notwithstanding.

But the patient rarely receives the emotional support he needs. Instead, he is primarily seen as a subject to be processed, a disease inside a human skin, an interesting diagnostic or scientific problem, good teaching material or whatever you will. He is manipulated, percussed, palpated, cut into, connected to tubes, swabbed, exhibited, wrapped, trundled from one white-coated person to another, all of whom are conversing in a cryptic jargon of vaguely reassuring phrases, right along the medical assembly (or disassembly) line. The patient has been depersonalised, estranged and alienated. It is true, of course, that the problem of alienation is endemic in industrial society. But the patient is victim to an alienation of a special kind, which vastly exceeds anything that has been noted among members of the work force, because it is magnified by association with illness and with anxiety related to pain and, perhaps, death. The patient is the forgotten man of medicine.

"The degradation of physicians in Germany exemplifies the decline and fall of a group whose moral obligations went by default in a single generation. The house would not have fallen had not many of the timbers been rotten. Descent into gas chambers by doctors of infamy had its beginnings *in disregard for patients.* The patient, however humble, and however ill, in whatever degree derelict and forlorn, has sacred rights."[1] It is these rights that are neglected by the medical practitioner in South Africa today.

Traditionally, the general practitioner has been the one medical professional with whom the patient can establish a relationship of intimacy outside the family. It is he who has been responsible for primary care, continuity of care, and reassurance to the patient: in short, for the essentials of adequate care. Sickness, by its very nature, gives rise to the need for compassionate care, and the specialist, even though he has had the standard medical training of all

1. Bean, W. B.: *J. of Lab. & Clin. med.,* 1952, 39, p. 3 (my italics).

doctors, is neither prepared nor equipped to provide it. Only the family doctor is in a position to do this; only he can steer the patient through the intricasies of the medical system with the minimum of bother and barriers, directing him to the appropriate facilities and the specialists who can help him best; and only he can oversee the general well-being of the patient.

In an earlier era the general practitioner was at the centre of the medical stage, constituting almost the totality of the fraternity's contingent. Although he was a specialist relative to other members of the community, he was a generalist in medicine and provided nearly the entire gamut of medical services. Today, general practitioners form only a small fraction of those working in the medical field, and fewer and fewer medical graduates are entering that sector. In 1931 four-fifths of all American doctors were in general practice; in 1966 three-quarters of them were in speciality practice, and the complete specialisation of doctors within another fifteen to twenty years has been forecast. General and unspecialised practice proffers no gleaming intellectual nuggets to bright, scientifically oriented medical students; they have far more spectacular things to do with their clever little minds. And no one with an iota of sense would ignore the lure of the income and other rewards some specialists are able to garner and display. Nor is the unfettered indulgence of five o'clock medicine inconsequential. Nowadays even obstetricians can guarantee their freedom in the evening and over the weekend by the appropriate management of the birth process. At least one gynaecologist in Johannesburg induces *all* his babies: "This is because I like them born during the day, when I and the nursing staff are operating at top efficiency. I choose a day convenient for the mother-to-be and her household, and I initiate labour."[1] Social induction by medical fiat. Mirror, mirror, on the wall, who's the sickest of us all? Well, at least the shrewd young doctor of tomorrow has *his* priorities all straightened out, and the delivery of health services, like the delivery of babies and the interests of the patient, is right down there at the bottom of his professional totem pole.

Unfortunately, the disappearance of the general practitioner through specialisation means a further and very critical decrease in the number of shock absorbers for human problems, which may

1. Garbett, S.: Report. *Star,* 5 March, 1976.

gravely disturb the emotional balance of society. The marked, and oft remarked, ambivalence of the public toward medicine and the medical profession is a very clear indication of the imminence of such a dislocation. The precarious equilibrium among the members of the medical species is out of kilter, sending through the social milieu ripples which have swelled into a tidal wave that very few may be able to weather.

For eons the brotherhood of healers has had a mandate from society to care for the health of the people. This mandated task of care involves both efficiency of treatment and compassion toward the patient. To the degree to which the medical care system fails to provide the supportive element, the package it spawns is unsatisfactory and, eventually, will be rejected out of hand. At this moment in time the chasm between the humanitarian - Hippocratic - and scientific - technocratic - aspects of medicine yawns perilously. Between these two cultures of contemporary medicine, I believe, the balance of the doctor-patient relationship has been upset not merely to the point of dysfunction; that was accomplished along with the lowering in status of the general practitioner. Now it has reached the point of full-fledged revolt by those who are outraged by and will no longer tolerate of any doctor actions and attitudes which negate his fiduciary commitment; a commitment, incidentally, which also implies that medicine will police its own house in return for the free hand society grants it in most professional matters.

This freedom from outside control rests on the claim that the practice of medicine is of such a complicated technical nature that laymen are unable to regulate or evaluate it intelligently. This attitude is at present echoed by our legal system. It is based on the further assertions that practitioners are trained to be responsible and have no need of supervision to perform at a competent or ethical level, and that proper regulatory action can be entrusted to the profession itself in the event of a practitioner proving not to be responsible. But the doctor's interactions with his patient are characterised by their total lack of visibility; they are subterranean, and no diviner-physician has been allotted the task of unearthing any buried infamy.

These lacunae inevitably lead to a casual attitude toward strictly proper conduct. If detection is unlikely, which it undeniably is, all the doctor has to do is satisfy his own conscience. While this is no doubt an effective restraint sometimes, or even most of the time, it can all too easily be circumvented by self-deception. The bluff "Nothing to worry about - a chance in a thousand", and a hundred-and-one similar utterances, are contumely, and satisfy neither the patient nor the rigours of ethics.

The distance between the patient and the doctor, the failure in communication and the lack of empathy has had a drastic and damaging impact on the medical enterprise. Something must be done to redress the current imbalance in the doctor-patient relationship. Neither litigation nor increasingly stringent regulatory measures can truly heal the wound. They can enforce a greater degree of equity, but they offer no solution to the tragic impasse we face in this sphere of human relationships.

Until one is found, what is there for the patient at a time when the medical profession's neglect of and disregard for his needs and rights have reached an all-time high? Many patients have responded to this medical felony by deserting the high road of orthodox medicine for the back alleys of unorthodox alternatives: chiropractors, homeopaths, naturopaths, and so forth, in so far as these people are still allowed to prey on the public. In South Africa, largely on the initiative of doctors, they have been legislated against to the point of virtual extinction. However, whichever of these avenues you explore, it is the doctor - or what he regards as his quack cousin, many times removed - who is held to be responsible for the cure, and not the patient. And yet the vast majority of ills, and even tissue pathology which is "incurable", are not beyond subjective control. They are, or at least they could be, a matter of responsibility for each individual, and we, as patients, *must* recognise them as such.

The critical question is how one can learn to assume responsibility for one's personal well-being in illness as well as in health. The notion that God helps those who help themselves is as old as the capitalistic ethic, but the injunction to the patient to "heal thyself" is relatively novel. It has little hope of consummation without some technique to encourage the active participation of the individual in both the prevention and treatment of breakdown in mental and physical processes.

Quite obviously no layman *can* acquire more than a cursory acquaintance of medical technology. The most he can hope for is an intelligent understanding of scientific progress on the medical front, so that he can make informed decisions about what is done with his body by the doctor. There is a great need for some service to the patient to help him make these decisions, perhaps in the form of a single journal devoted to this purpose, rather than the odd articles dispersed throughout the popular weeklies.

Nevertheless, the current inaccessibility of scientific information because of its unassimilable presentation in no way prevents him from taking an active part in maintaining his personal well-being. There are two clear-cut aspects to health care, and the most critical of these, that concerning the patient's emotional well-being, is certainly amenable to influence by the individual himself. This is due to the phenomenal development recently of the experimental psychology of learning, which seriously challenges the modern concept that the doctor is solely responsible for the cure, with the patient a passive recipient of, rather than an active participant in, therapy.

The story of psychology since its divorce from philosophy at the start of this century is largely the story of the expansion of the theory of learning, and there have been sufficient gains in this area, and in related areas inside and outside the discipline, to formulate a therapeutic principle that holds rich promise. At its base is a behavioural control mechanism called biofeedback, by means of which the patient can, for the first time, take an active role in literally learning not to be sick.

Biofeedback involves the use of bioelectric monitoring instruments such as the electromyogram (EMG) to detect and amplify autonomic (or involuntary), as well as neural processes within the body, and to feed this information back to the individual in some concrete form. Thus, for example, a person with a tension headache (tension headaches are caused by abnormal levels of tension or contraction in certain muscles of the head) can ascertain the level of tension through the use of the EMG. The amplification and display system which is part of the monitoring equipment enables him to "hear" the level of muscular activity as a series of small clicks that are spaced in time, almost as the air pressure gauge at a service station indicates tyre pressure by means of clicks. Alternatively, he can "see" the level of tension by reading a dial. Recording techniques of this nature enable the individual to gain control over his autonomic nervous system, and thus over his emotional performance.

The clicks that the person hears, or the light that he sees on the display panel, are sensory signals, feedback from his autonomic nervous system, that inform him of how well he is doing in his attempt to bring that specific involuntary function under voluntary self-control. The feedback indicates to him minute quanta of early success in changing the working of an autonomic function in a desired direction. Gradually, through a process of trial and error, the person learns to control the feedback and, consequently, his inner reaction system. As he becomes more successful, he learns to associate certain thoughts, as well as internal sensations, however subtle, with changes in the feedback he sees, and this enhances the transfer of the control strategies that he acquires in the clinic or laboratory to real-life situations.

Biofeedback or autonomic learning is a procedure that provides the patient with a potential means of preventing illness or curing himself by helping him to regulate the pace of his daily life style, of his thought patterns and body processes, hopefully reducing his susceptibility to pathologic levels of hyperactivation when he is faced with stressful life events.

Contemporary psychology, therefore, holds out hope to those many who have been denied it by members of the medical profession. At a time when man's alienation from self and from others is one of industrial society's most enduring and poignant problems, when for many life has lost its essential meaning and when the helping professions, and most particularly the doctors, care next to nothing – in some cases, nothing at all – about humanity, there is one small ray of light on the horizon: a means whereby the individual can take matters into his own hands and fight, and win, the good fight.

Appendices

I   The Case

1. Summary: Medical Chronology

22 October, 1974:	Dr. Davids.
20 December, 1974:	Dr. Green – first visit.
20 December, 1974:	X-ray of cervical and head region; comprehensive blood tests.
8 January, 1975:	Myasthenia exclusion tests.
22 January, 1975:	Dr. Green – second visit.
28 January, 1975:	Myelogram.
14 February, 1975:	Dr. Green – third visit.
17 February, 1975:	First EEG.
18 February, 1975:	Brain scan.
3 March, 1975:	Dr. Green – fourth visit.
7 April, 1975:	Second EEG.
8 April, 1975:	Dr. Green – fifth visit.
3 May, 1975:	Third EEG.
25 June, 1975:	Fourth EEG.
7 July, 1975:	Dr. Green – sixth visit.
15 July, 1975:	Angiogram and curare test.
13 August, 1975:	Dr. Rice.
26 September, 1975:	Dr. Green – seventh visit.
27 September, 1975:	Rescreen of myelogram and removal of Myodil.
14 November, 1975:	Professor Barron.
15 November, 1975:	Dr. Green – eighth visit.
18 November, 1975:	Mr. Kenny – first visit.
10 December, 1975:	Dr. Bell.
18 December, 1975:	Dr. Evans – first visit.
24 December, 1975:	Mr. Kenny – second visit.

2. Summary: Symptomatology

October 1973 – January 1975: Excessive fatigue in lower limbs; difficulty in walking. Pain in right knee. "Giving" in right knee and dragging of right leg.

October 1973 – June 1975: Emotional apathy.

October 1973 – June 1975: Euphoria.

January 1974 – January 1975; December 1975: Double vision; patchy vision; blurring of right eye.

January 1974 – January 1975: Weakness in upper limbs. Trembling in right hand.

January 1974 – March 1975: Daily spasms and cramp in right leg.

September 1974 – April 1975: Fits.

March 1975 – February 1976: Ptosis of right eye. Constriction of right pupil. Occasional recurrences after February 1976.

March 1975 – April 1975: Fainting.

February 1975 – March 1975: Spasm of trunk on left side.

February 1975 – : Difficulties with speech.

March 1975: Total hearing loss on several occasions.

March 1975 – : Partial hearing loss.

April 1975 – July 1975: Severe spasms in upper right arm and shoulder. Occasional concomitant spasms in right side of face. Dilation of right pupil and constriction of left. Return of excessive fatigue.

July 1975 – September 1975: Lameness of right leg. Pain in lower back. Pain in right leg. Severe pins and needles in hands and feet.

July 1975 – : "Burn" and pain: lower back and right leg.

August 1975 – : "Burn": lower back and right leg; involvement of left leg.

September 1975 – : Occasional inability to walk. Limping to greater or lesser extent.

December 1975: Acute vertigo; severe multiple bruising and injury to nose and ear during fits.

3. Radiologist's Report: Myelogram

28th January, 1975

6 cc of Myodil were introduced by lumbar puncture. The entire thecal space was examined but particular attention was paid to the cervical region. The contrast medium flowed freely and easily showing no obstruction, holdup or deformity at any point. The width of the cervical cord appeared normal.

Films obtained during screening include shoot through lateral views and confirm the normal appearances in the cervical region.

The patient was then placed supine and the contrast medium induced to run into the cistern magna. The impressions of both tonsils were clearly seen. The right tonsil was seen to be lobulated and the lower lobule was well engaged in the foramen magnum. The left tonsil was in normal position.

The films obtained confirm the findings described.

Comment: Cervical myelography has shown no pathology in this region. P.F.C. has shown the right tonsil to consist of two lobules with a small inferior lobule well engaged in the foramen magnum. The left tonsil is in normal position.

4. Myelogram

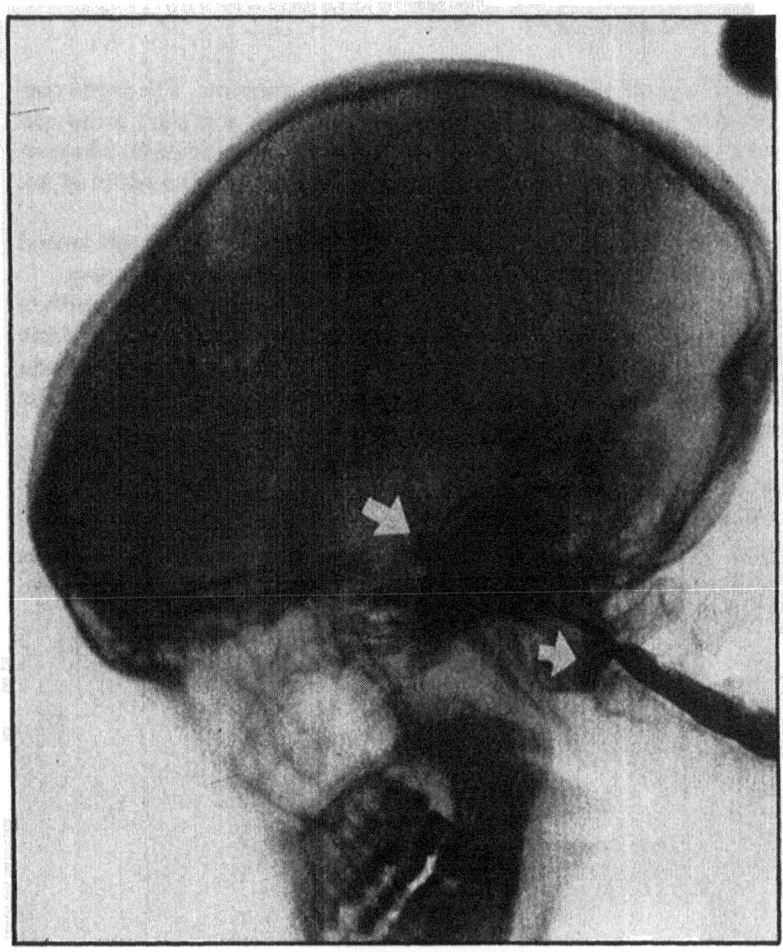

Myelogram 28.1.1975. Passage of Myodil along spinal cord, and entry into skull. Arrow above Myodil indicates earring. Jewelry is not usually worn during radiography. However, the patient entering Lords Nursing Home is well advised to expect the unexpected.

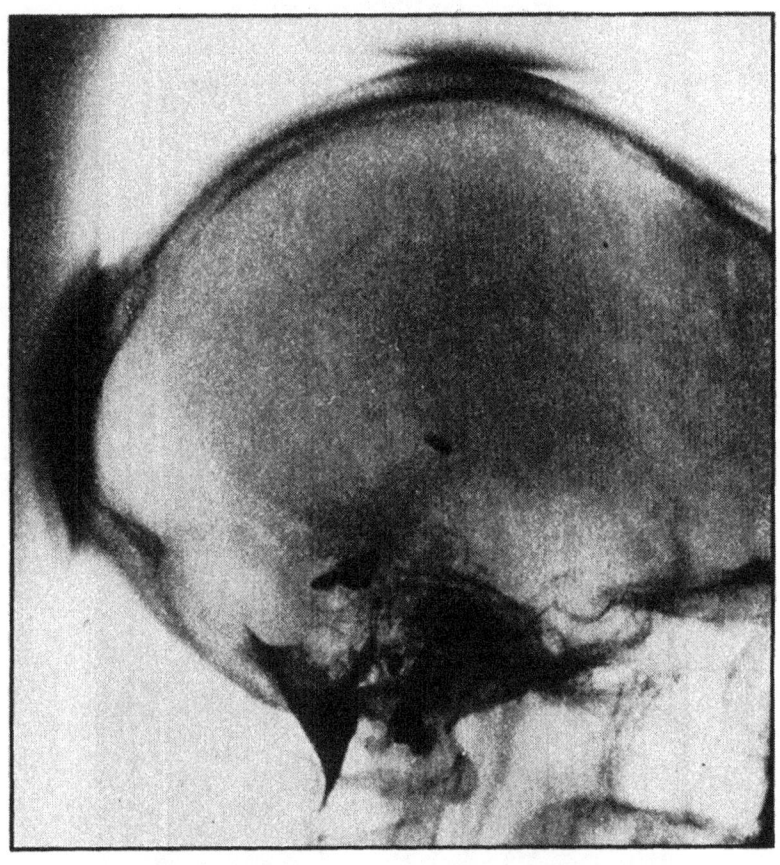

Myelogram 28.1.1975. The cerebellar tonsil (clarified by the Myodil) which was diagnosed by Dr Green as an Arnold-Chiari malformation. It must be pointed out, however, that diagnosis also includes the clinical picture.

Dispersed globules of Myodil also appear here.

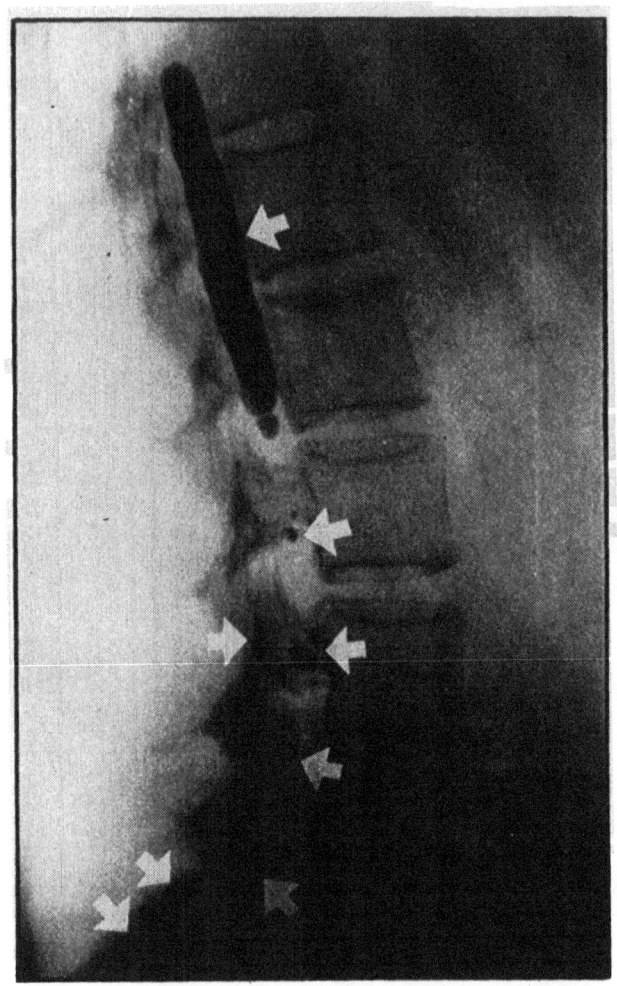

X-ray plate taken by Dr Peters of lower lumbar region on 3.9.1975. The arrows indicate:
1. The Myodil which remained in the spine after its introduction for purposes of diagnosis on 28.1.1975. This was removed on 26.9.1975.
2. Particles or globules of Myodil dispersed along spinal cord which cannot be removed and which can, and in my case did, cause arachnoiditis (see p. 134 of text).

5. EEG Reports

17th February, 1975

The EEG was abnormal due to:

1. considerable, generalised, low voltage 18 Hz activity;
2. numerous focal independently left and right temporal and post temporal beta paroxysms and 3, 4 and 6 Hz runs, the latter augmented on the left and the former diffused by hyperventilation.

The EEG suggests a dysfunction, probably related to cortical damage, of the left temporal and post temporal areas, with centrencephalic involvement. A repeat after about 6 weeks is suggested.

7th April, 1975

The EEG remains abnormal due to numerous left hemisphere runs and bursts of low voltage sharp wave and beta activity, both augmented by photic stimulation and hyperventilation, with focal left post temporal components. Comparable right-sided activity was seen less frequently.

The EEG shows little change since that of 17th February 1975, and remains suggestive of a left post temporal dysfunction, perhaps epileptogenic, with centrencephalic involvement.

Regular repeat EEGs are suggested.

14th May, 1975

The EEG remains abnormal due to:

1. excessive generalized low voltage beta activity, appearing also on eye opening and in independent left- and right-sided bursts during photic stimulation, and augmented by photic stimulation and hyperventilation;
2. numerous focal medium-low voltage spikes in the left fronto-temporal area during rest, photic stimulation and hyperventilation;
3. medium-low voltage 5 and 6 Hz runs in the left temporal region, augmented by hyperventilation;

4. dubious slow (2 and 3 Hz) wave activity in the left frontal and post temporal areas during hyperventilation.

The EEG suggests a left fronto-temporal epileptogenic dysfunction. The record shows noteworthy deterioration since that of 7 April, 1975, due to the appearance of spike and 5 and 6 Hz activity, and possibly, 2 and 3 Hz activity, in the left temporal circumference. These features give rise to the possibility of a cerebral lesion, and suggest the continuation of EEGs at six-week intervals.

25th June, 1975

The EEG remains abnormal due to:

1. very considerable low and medium voltage spike, sharp, beta and slow wave (3 to 6 Hz) activity in the left posterior area, often focal in the left post temporal region and markedly augmented by photic stimulation and hyperventilation;
2. excessive generalised low voltage beta activity, augmented by photic stimulation and hyperventilation;
3. pronounced interhemispheric asymmetry and asynchrony.

Photic stimulation and hyperventilation both induced subjective feelings of unpleasantness and left posterior headache and pressure.

The EEG has deteriorated further since that of 14 May, 1975, and is strongly suggestive of a left post temporal dysfunction, possibly epileptogenic, although the increase in slow activity may indicate an organic involvement. In view of the further EEG deterioration and the correlation of clinical and EEG signs further neurological investigation would appear advised. Follow up EEGs should be continued.

6. Radiologist's Report: Rescreen of Myelogram

27th September, 1975

1. Contrast medium flowed freely and easily showing no obstruction, holdup or deformity at any point.

2. The region from L1 to L5 was examined and no abnormality was noted in this region.

3. The films obtained during screening confirmed the absence of any abnormalities.

Comment: Lumbar myelography has revealed no lesion in relation to the thecal space in this region.

7. Correspondence

Letter to Green on subject of phone calls,
5th November, 1975

It is impossible to contact you by telephone. Approximately 3 months ago, and subsequently, the ladies at your switchboard refused me access to yourself. I have during these 3 months been obliged to apply for sick leave. My period of absence has now expired and I judge the medical situation – neurological or otherwise – to have deteriorated. I appreciate that you were present on Saturday, September 27, when the myodil was removed, but apart from temporary relief, this has had no effect.

The general physician attending me has done all he can to alleviate the situation. However, I am experiencing considerably more pain than you apparently realise. My husband, unfortunately, has been obliged to witness most of it. I deeply resent, therefore, your unwillingness as my specialist to be available and to offer reassurance to him when it is most necessary.

Green's reply, 6th November, 1975

Thank you for your letter of 5.11.75.

I really must take you to task.

It is by no means impossible to contact me by telephone. Had you phoned yourself I would have spoken to you. On the day that your husband phoned I had already spent some time talking to your house doctor and had arranged for a consultation to take place with

Professor Barron. There was therefore no need for me to speak to him in the middle of a busy consulting time.

I reiterate, had you phoned yourself with a valid complaint then I would have found the time to speak to you and done all I could to help you. As it was I had no idea that you still had pain because I had not heard from you.

I have now spoken to Professor Barron and he has agreed to see you any time in the next week or so. All you have to do is phone him one evening and he will make the necessary arrangements. He is fully conversant with the facts of your case.

II Medical Ethics

The traditional code of medical ethics is enshrined in the Hippocratic Oath. After World War II the World Medical Association condemned the crimes and the inhuman acts committed by German physicians and adopted a modern version of the Hippocratic Oath at its Second General Assembly in Geneva in 1948. Known as the Declaration of Geneva, it is a pledge intended to be made by a medical practitioner at the time of being admitted as a member of the medical profession.

1. The Declaration of Geneva

I solemnly pledge myself to consecrate my life to the service of humanity;

I will give to my teachers the respect and gratitude which is their due;

I will practice my profession with conscience and dignity;

The health of my patient will be my first consideration;

I will respect the secrets which are confided in me;

I will maintain by all the means in my power, the honour and the noble traditions of the medical profession;

My colleagues will be my brothers;

I will not permit considerations of religion, nationality, race, party politics or social standing to intervene between my duty and my patient;

I will maintain the utmost respect for human life, from the time of conception; even under threat, I will not use my medical knowledge contrary to the laws of humanity.

I make these promises solemnly, freely and upon my honor.

165

2. International Code of Medical Ethics

At the Third General Assembly of the World Medical Association held in London in October 1949, an International Code of Medical Ethics was adopted. The Medical Association of South Africa is a member of the World Medical Association and therefore subscribes to the Code.

Duties of Doctors in General

A doctor must always maintain the highest standards of professional conduct.

A doctor must practice his profession uninfluenced by motives of profit.

The following practices are deemed unethical:
1. Any self advertisement except such as is expressly authorised by the national code of medical ethics.
2. Collaboration in any form of medical service in which the doctor does not have professional independence.
3. Receiving any money in connection with services rendered to a patient other than a proper professional fee, even with the knowledge of a patient.

Any act, or advice which would weaken physical or mental resistance of a human being may be used only in his interest.

A doctor is advised to use great caution in divulging discoveries or new techniques of treatment.

A doctor should certify or testify only to that which he has personally verified.

Duties of Doctors to the Sick

A doctor must always bear in mind the obligation of preserving human life.

A doctor owes to his patient complete loyalty and all the resources of his science. Whenever an examination or treatment is beyond his capacity he should summon another doctor who has the necessary ability.

A doctor shall preserve absolute secrecy on all he knows about his patient because of the confidence entrusted in him.

A doctor must give emergency care as a humanitarian duty unless he is assured that others are willing and able to give such care.

Duties of Doctors to Each Other

A doctor ought to behave to his colleagues as he would have them behave to him.

A doctor must not entice patients from his colleagues.

A doctor must observe the principles of *The Declaration of Geneva* approved by The World Medical Association.

III   Postscript

Letter from Green,
19th February, 1976

I was phoned today by Dr. James of the research institute who told me that you asked to see the EEG which had been done on you. I saw no objection to this, and have given him carte blanche in showing you the reports and the EEGs.

He has told me that you are busy collecting "Evidence" whatever that means. I understand that you are writing a book.

I think I would like it on record that at no time did I ever entertain a diagnosis of disseminated sclerosis in your symptoms and signs, and even now when other doctors have told you that you do have disseminated sclerosis, I just cannot agree with them. I have never seen anybody with disseminated sclerosis present with the myriad signs and symptoms which you have, and while I am prepared to go so far as to say I am not quite sure what the specific diagnosis is, I will also put my neck out and say that in my opinion you do not have disseminated sclerosis. I have said as much to Mr. Kenny and to Dr. Rice, which you can confirm by phoning either of them.

I hope you are settling down, but if you have any further problems I will of course be delighted to discuss them with you.

Epilogue

There are some people, and I am one of them, for whom the search for the truth is the most fascinating and worth-while quest of all. Obviously, a large query in my life is the truth of my own condition. Under ordinary circumstances I would be willing to undergo any reasonable test or examination, regardless of the risks involved, to resolve - finally - this question.

However, I believe - and the reader must form his own judgment concerning the validity of this belief - that my mind and my body have been wantonly, even brutally, abused by some medical practitioners who care neither for the truth, nor for the integrity of the human body, nor for the psychological reality of the human mind.

I cannot undo what has been done; nor do I really see how the medical profession could make reparation for its collective guilt. Moreover, there is as yet no indication of any means of overcoming the pain that is now an intrinsic part of my daily life. That I shall do so is, however, beyond doubt. My absolute faith in the infinite ingenuity of the human mind remains intact.

Nevertheless, I have reached the point when I must take whatever steps are open to me to prevent the further abuse of my body should I be rendered incapable of protecting myself.

The human being is at his most vulnerable at birth, and in the presence of death. Between these two points, the great challenge, the very purpose of existence, its *raison d'être,* is to conquer - in a degree appropriate to each stage of development, and without denial of the rights of others - the vicissitudes of life. This I will continue to do to the best of my ability. But since death, like incurable disease, is no longer an empty abstraction for me - if only because I have passed the half-way mark - the following document has been given legal effect.

169

To My Family and General Practitioner

This Declaration is made by me, Cynthia Fay Birrer, at a time when I am of sound mind and after careful consideration.

If the time comes when I can no longer take part in decisions for my own future, let this Declaration stand as the testament to my wishes:

1. If there is no reasonable prospect of my recovery from the physical illness or impairment which causes me severe distress and which may render me incapable of rational existence, I request that I be allowed to die and not be kept alive by artificial means, and that I receive whatever quantity of drugs may be required to keep me *free* from pain or distress even if the moment of death is hastened.

2. I further request that if it is not possible to keep me free from pain, that I receive a sufficient quantity of drugs to hasten death.

3. I expressly forbid an autopsy.

This declaration is signed and dated by me in the presence of the two undermentioned witnesses present at the same time who, at my request, in my presence and in the presence of each other, have hereunto subscribed their names as witnesses.

Johannesburg,
July, 1976

170

Bibliography

Alfidi, R. J.: "Informed consent. A study of patient reaction". *J.A.M.A.*, 216:1325, 1971.

Belli, M.: *Ready for the Plaintiff.* New York, Charter Books, 1956.

Bergen, R. P.: "Medical arbitration experiments". *J.A.M.A.*, 211:351, 1970.

Bergen, R. P.: "Mediation of liability claims". *J.A.M.A., 222:241, 1972.*

Blom, S.: "Tic douloureux treated with new anti-convulsant; experiences with G32883". *Arch Neurol.*, 9:285, 1963.

Brain, Lord and Walton, J.N.: *Brain's Diseases of the Nervous System.* London, Oxford University Press, 1969.

Breuer, J. and Freud, S.: *Studies on Hysteria.* New York, Basic Books, 1957.

Curran, W. J.: "Focus on medical malpractice – some alternative plans for compensation". *New Engl. J. Med.*, 286:987, 1972.

Currie, S.: *The Yorkshire Post News Service,* 27 January, 1976.

Currie, S., Heathfield, K.W.G., Henson, R.A. and Scott, D. F.: "Clinical course and prognosis of temporal lobe epilepsy". *Brain,* 94:173, 1971.

Davies, F. L.: "Effect of unabsorbed radiographic contrast media on the central nervous system". *Lancet,* 15:11, 1956.

Dukeminier, J. and Sanders, D.: "Organ transplantation". *New Engl. J. Med.,* 279: 414, 1968.

"Ethical Guidelines for organ transplantation". *J.A.M.A.,* 205:341, 1968.

FDA Drug Bulletin, October, 1972.

French, J. D.: "Clinical manifestations of lumbar spinal arachnoiditis. A report of thirteen cases". *Surgery,* 20:718, 1946.

Garbett, S.: Report. *Star,* 5 March, 1976.

Garrison, F. H.: *An Introduction to the History of Medicine.* Philadelphia, W. B. Saunders Co., 1921.

Holder, A. R.: "Joint screening panels". *J.A.M.A.,* 215:1715, 1971.

Holder, A. R.: "Physician's liability for adverse drug reactions". *J.A.M.A.,* 213:2143, 1970.

Hurteau, E. F., Baird, W. C. and Sinclair, E.: "Arachnoiditis following use of iodised oil". *J. Bone Joint Surg.,* 36A:393, 1954.

Ingelfinger, F. J.: "Informed (but uneducated) consent". *New Engl. J. Med.,* 287:465, 1972.

Janet, P.: *Principles of Psychotherapy.* New York, MacMillan, 1924.

171

Katz, J.: *Experimentation with Human Beings*. New York, Russell Sage, 1973.

Klass, A.: *There's Gold in Them Thar Pills*. London, Penguin Books, 1975.

Mason, M. S. and Raaf, J.: "Complications of Pantopaque myelography: Case Report and review". *J. Neurosurg.*, 19:302, 1962.

Mills, D. H.: "Whither informed consent?" *J.A.M.A.*, 229:305, 1974.

Modlin, H. C.: "The physician and the legal system". *J.A.M.A.*, 221: 1387, 1972.

Nathan, H. L.: *Medical Negligence: Legal Case Studies*. London, Butterworth, 1957.

McAlpine, D., Lumsden, C. E. and Acheson, E. D.: *Multiple Sclerosis*. Edinburgh, E. & S. Livingstone Ltd., 1965.

Patterson, R. H. Jr., Goodell, H. and Dunning, H. S.: "Complications of carotid angiography". *Arch. Neurol.*, 10:513, 1964.

Peacher, W. G. and Robertson, R. C. L.: "Pantopaque myelography: results, comparison of contrast media and spinal fluid reaction". *J. Neurosurg*, 2:220, 1945.

Petito, F. and Plum, F.: "The lumbar puncture". *New Engl. J. Med.*, 290:225, 1974.

Ramsey, G. H., French, J. D. and Strain, W. H.: "Iodinated organic compounds as contrast media for radiographic diagnoses". *Radiology*, 43:236, 1944.

Sjostr̈om, H. and Nilsson, R.: *Thalidomide and the Power of the Drug Companies*. London, Penguin Books, 1972.

Stetler, J. and Moritz, A. R.: *Doctor and Patient and the Law*. St. Louis, Mosby Co., 1971.

Strauss, S.A.: "The legal remedy which is a medical nightmare". *Codicillus*, 8, 1966.

Strauss, S.A.: "The physician's liability for malpractice: a fair solution to the problem of proof?" *S.A. Law J.*, 419, 1967.

Strauss, S.A.: "Medical negligence. In Doctor & Law". *Documenta Geigy*, 4, 1969.

Strauss, S.A. and Strydom, M. J.: *Die Suid-Afrikaanse Geneeskundige Reg.* Pretoria, J. L. van Schaik, Bpk., 1967.